T0282315

This book provides a handy reference guide for medical practitioners who do not have specialist knowledge in paediatric audiology but who, nevertheless, will encounter many cases with mild hearing impairment in childhood and occasional cases with more severe hearing problems.

The test procedures used to assess the presence, type, nature and degree of hearing impairment are described with guidance on how to interpret the information provided in audiological reports.

A book of this nature is long overdue and its presence is very timely, given the appearance of various publications outlining requirements for improved quality and more effective service provision for hearing-impaired children. The early detection of hearing problems is of fundamental importance in childhood and the medical practitioner has a central and active role in this process. Guidance on what practitioners can and should do is given in the text, together with the answers to many questions that parents bring to the surgery.

THE MEDICAL PRACTITIONER'S
GUIDE TO
PAEDIATRIC AUDIOLOGY

THE MEDICAL PRACTITIONER'S GUIDE TO PAEDIATRIC AUDIOLOGY

Edited by

BARRY McCORMICK

*Children's Hearing Assessment Centre
Nottingham*

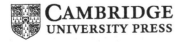

CAMBRIDGE
UNIVERSITY PRESS

Published by the Press Syndicate of the University of Cambridge
The Pitt Building, Trumpington Street, Cambridge CB2 1RP
40 West 20th Street, New York, NY 10011-4211, USA
10 Stamford Road, Oakleigh, Melbourne 3166, Australia

First published 1995

A catalogue record for this book is available from the British Library

Library of Congress cataloguing in publication data

The medical practitioners guide to paediatric audiology / Barry
McCormick (ed.).
    p. cm.
Includes index.
ISBN 0 521 45988 5 (pbk.)
1. Hearing disorders in children.   I. McCormick, Barry.
[DNLM: 1. Hearing Disorders – in infancy & childhood – handbooks.
2. Hearing Disorders – diagnosis – handbooks.   3. Hearing Aids – in
infancy & childhood – handbooks.   4. Hearing Tests – in infancy &
childhood – handbooks.   WV 39 M489   1995]
RF291.5.C45M43   1995
618.92'0978 – dc20
DNLM/DLC
for Library of Congress   94-36575 CIP

ISBN 0 521 45988 5 paperback

Transferred to digital printing 2003

WS

Thanks are expressed to
Kathryn Beardsley for
patiently typing the entire
script of this volume

Contents

Contents

Contributors

Yvonne Cope — Children's Hearing Assessment Centre, Ropewalk House, 113 The Ropewalk, Nottingham NG1 6HA, UK.

Catherine Cottingham — Children's Hearing Assessment Centre, Ropewalk House, 113 The Ropewalk, Nottingham NG1 6HA, UK.

Kevin P. Gibbin — Department of Otolaryngology, Queen's Medical Centre, University Hospital, Nottingham NG7 2UH, UK.

Nick Jones — Department of Otolaryngology, Queen's Medical Centre, University Hospital, Nottingham NG7 2UH, UK.

Barry McCormick — Children's Hearing Assessment Centre, Ropewalk House, 113 The Ropewalk, Nottingham NG1 6HA, UK.

Angela Maxwell — Children's Hearing Assessment Centre, Ropewalk House, 113 The Ropewalk, Nottingham NG1 6HA, UK.

Jackie Moon — Children's Hearing Assessment Centre, Ropewalk House, 113 The Ropewalk, Nottingham NG1 6HA, UK.

Susan Robinson — Children's Hearing Assessment Centre, Ropewalk House, 113 The Ropewalk, Nottingham NG1 6HA, UK.

Sarah Sheppard — Department of Experimental Psychology, University of Sussex, Falmer, Brighton BN1 9QG, UK.

Sally Wood — Children's Hearing Assessment Centre, Ropewalk House, 113 The Ropewalk, Nottingham NG1 6HA, UK.

Preface

The need for this book became apparent during a series of courses on child health surveillance on which the editor lectured to some 3000 medical practitioners over a 2 year period. The same questions arose repeatedly and it was clear that a basic text was needed, specifically to answer these questions at an appropriate level for non-specialist doctors who, nevertheless, have a significant and active role to play in helping to detect hearing problems. In the surgery parents' questions must be answered with insight and with awareness of the basic issues. They raise questions after ear, nose and throat (ENT) and audiological assessment sessions and they bring the terminology from those clinics, and from media coverage, into the doctor's surgery.

This book contains an introduction to paediatric audiology and addresses such questions as

Can hearing be tested in the newborn?
Can hearing aids and cochlear implants be supplied to babies before 3
 months of age?
How do you interpret a tympanogram?
Why is masking undertaken in audiometry?
What is the purpose of bone-conduction testing?
How can infants hear quiet sounds but not discriminate speech?
What is a bone-anchored hearing aid?
Can cochlear implants restore hearing to normal?
What happens after hearing aids have been supplied or after cochlear
 implant surgery?

The answers are contained in the following pages and it is hoped that this book will be of value to any doctor who comes into contact with hearing-impaired children.

B. McCormick
Nottingham

Acknowledgement

The editor acknowledges the help and support of the parents who have given permission for their children's photographs to be reproduced in this book.

1

Introduction to hearing problems in childhood

BARRY McCORMICK

Severe and profound hearing impairment is rare, affecting only one to two babies per thousand births. In nearly 50% of the cases no definite cause of deafness can be found but it is known that those born in special care units are ten times more likely to be affected than their well baby counterparts. Davis and Wood (1992) demonstrated in a group of 2000 babies in the UK that 70% of the hearing impaired from special care units had additional disabilities.

By the age of 3 years, 9% of the deaf population will acquire sensorineural or mixed losses and this proportion rises, eventually to 20%, in later childhood years. Many of these acquired losses will be profound or total in nature with meningitis being the single most common cause. Although this represents a small proportion of all hearing-impaired children it is a very significant group demanding diagnostic and rehabilitation resources and some may become candidates for cochlear implantation.

Another group requiring considerable resources is deaf children with additional disability and special care unit babies are nine times more likely to have dual or multiple disability. Of such cases from special care units, 43% have mixed (conductive and sensorineural) losses in early childhood and this is a much higher proportion than the 10% with mixed losses in the rest of the population. The prevalence of sensorineural hearing loss decreases with severity and a typical finding for the better ear hearing would be:

50–80 dBHL; 1 in 1000 infants
81–95 dBHL; 1 in 2000 infants
above 95 dBHL; 1 in 3500 infants

Conductive hearing losses are much more common and 6% of children will have an episode of significant conductive hearing loss (above

20 dB) at some stage. Most of these will occur below the age of 4 years and very rarely above the age of 8 years. About 80% of babies will have middle-ear fluid within the first year of life and the majority will require no treatment. It is, however, necessary to identify those where the fluid persists and causes a marked hearing problem. This topic is discussed in detail in Chapter 7.

It will be appreciated from the above introduction that, with the exception of persistent conductive hearing problems, hearing impairment in childhood is extremely rare. A practising doctor with 2000 registered patients will see 40 or so children per year with conductive hearing loss but only one severely/profoundly deaf child might appear in 20 years of practice.

The impact of deafness on child development

Severe and profound deafness can affect a child's social, emotional, intellectual and linguistic development. The earlier it is detected and compensated for with appropriate hearing aid provision or the introduction of a manual system of communication, the less will be the adverse impact on later development. No hearing aid can restore hearing to undistorted normal levels.

Early detection is particularly crucial in congenitally deaf babies so that the early stage of neural plasticity can be harnessed, with the use of hearing aids and/or a signing system, to assist the process of speech and language development by establishing the necessary neural pathways. The days of assuming that speech and language start with the first words at 12–18 months are far gone and we now know that even in the first weeks of life the infant is exposed to important auditory experience, which forms the foundation for later speech and language development. If the early sensitive stages for language development are missed, as is the case with late-detected hearing problems, it can be expected that there will be serious consequences and the child will be prevented from achieving full linguistic potential. Late detection is anything beyond the first months of life. The average age of detection of hearing loss in excess of 50 dB is 3 years in the USA (NIH Consensus Statement, 1993) and 2 years in the UK (Davis and Sancho, 1988) and this is not a satisfactory situation, given that good screening tests can be applied within the first year.

The medical practitioner has a responsibility to ensure that thorough investigations are made if there is any evidence for, or suspicion of, a hearing problem. Parents are normally correct if they suspect the presence of a hearing disorder and the practitioner is advised to take such suspicion seriously. Parents are now exercising rights on behalf of their children, some of which may lead to litigation claims against any professional who delays access to help and treatment. Techniques are now available for testing the hearing of babies at any stage, including within the first days of life and hence no child is too young to be referred for investigation and no child is too young to be considered for the fitting of hearing aids given that it normally takes a few weeks for hearing investigations to be completed at the diagnostic level. Figure 1.1 shows a baby wearing appropriate hearing aids.

It has already been stated that not all hearing problems are severe or profound and not all are permanent. Some children will be disadvantaged by temporary fluctuating losses resulting from otitis media. The inconsistency of auditory input from the fluctuations will add to the problem of loss of hearing sensitivity. Each 10 dB drop in hearing level corresponds to a halving of the subjective loudness and although losses of 20–40 dB may be termed minor or moderate, and might be tolerated by an adult, the effects are far from mild for infants during the forma-

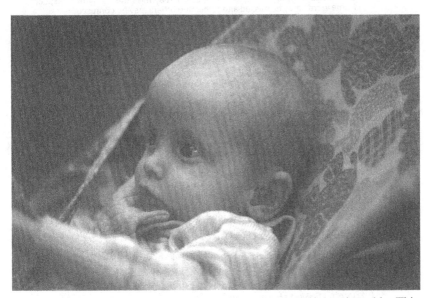

Figure 1.1. A baby wearing miniature postaural hearing aids. This child was fitted with hearing aids at the early age of 10 weeks, despite the fact that he was 11 weeks premature.

4   *B. McCormick*

tive stages of language development. Figure 1.2 shows the author's
advice sheet to help parents and teachers to understand such cases.

Another type of hearing loss that can lead to inconsistency of input,
and to lack of understanding by parents, is high tone sensorineural dis-

4

C.H.A.C. 4

NOTTINGHAMSHIRE CHILDREN'S HEARING ASSESSMENT CENTRE
ADVISORY DOCUMENT No. 2

ADVICE FOR PARENTS AND TEACHERS
CONCERNING CHILDREN WITH HEARING PROBLEMS
OF A MINOR DEGREE

A child with a slight hearing problem may not need or even be able to benefit
from a hearing aid but, nevertheless, he or she may be at risk both in terms of
language development and in terms of educational progess. It is hoped that the
advice given below will help parents and teachers to form some appreciation of the
nature of the child's problems and this may help to lessen the risk to the child.

The Child's Problems

1. It is important to understand that the child's main problem is not lack of
   awareness of sound for in certain circumstances even very quiet sounds may be
   heard. The problem is more one of sound confusion because some parts of
   speech may be heard less well than others. The child may be aware of a very
   quiet voice or even a whisper but he or she may miss the clarity of the speech.
   Some words may be missed altogether and others may be confused.

2. It is highly likely that a child with this degree of hearing disorder will have been
   accused of being rather slow or inattentive when in fact the child has a genuine
   problem in making sense of what is said.

3. The child's problem will be much greater in noisy surroundings or in situations
   where more than one person is speaking at the same time.

4. The hearing levels may fluctuate from day to day. On good days the child's
   hearing may appear to be virtually normal and on poor days the child may have
   considerable difficulty.

5. If one ear is affected more than the other the child may experience difficulty in
   locating sounds and in understanding speech presented on the poor side.

What Parents and Teachers Should Do

1. Careful thought should be given to seating arrangements in classrooms or to the
   distance at which speech is presented to the child in other situations. The
   speaker should attempt to be as near as possible to the child and be on the
   better side if one ear is affected more than the other.

2. The child will be helped if he or she can see the speaker's face.

3. Patience may be needed if the child repeatedly misunderstands.

Dr. B. McCormick PhD, BSc, Cert. T. Deaf, Dip. Audiol.
Director of the Children's Hearing Assessment Centre.

Figure 1.2. The author's advice sheet concerning children with minor
degrees of hearing loss.

orders. In such cases low and middle frequencies in the speech frequency range may not be heard at all. The affected child will respond to quiet sounds but may not be able to make sense of speech because the high frequency consonant sounds, which give meaning and intelligibility to speech, may be absent. This type of hearing loss can be detected only if tests incorporating specific high frequency stimuli are used. Such tests will be described in this book.

The possibility that a child might feign deafness as an attention seeking strategy should not be overlooked. This form of behaviour is not uncommon, particularly in girls around the age of 8 years and above and they can be very convincing to the extent that hearing aids may be requested. Skilled audiological testing is required to detect non-organic hearing loss of this nature and the clinician is usually alerted to the possibility that such a condition might be present when a child's performance in a speech discrimination test of hearing is better than would be expected from the audiometric thresholds. True hysterical conversion deafness is extremely rare and virtually unknown in children. The pattern observed is usually one of feigning or malingering but the psychological motive for such behaviour may need to be investigated with considerable tact and sensitivity.

How to aid detection

It has already been stated that parents are a valuable resource in the early detection process and the first recommendation to the medical practitioner is '**Listen to the parents and act upon their suspicions**'. The author's 'Can your baby hear you?' checklist (Figure 1.3) can aid this process.

The second recommendation is '**If in doubt, refer**'. Parents do not notice all kinds of deafness and high tone deafness is the classical one that will be missed if good testing is not undertaken to exclude it. In the absence of good testing such cases may be detected at a late stage when speech and language delay become apparent and often with accompanying behaviour disturbance and attention problems. By then much harm will have been done. Such problems can be avoided by including a high tone test stimulus in a neonatal hearing screening test or in the Distraction Test (McCormick, 1991). The Distraction Test has been shown to be a valid test within a community context, when performed well (McCormick, 1983) and Davis and Wood (1992) showed that in one district 72% of babies with losses greater than 50 dBHL were

Hints for Parents ———————————————————————

"Can your baby hear you?"

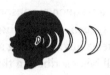

Here is a checklist of some of the general signs you can look for in your baby's first year:-

YES/NO

Shortly after birth
Your baby should be startled by a sudden loud noise such as a hand clap or a door slamming and should blink or open his eyes widely to such sounds.

By 1 Month
Your baby should be beginning to notice sudden prolonged sounds like the noise of a vacuum cleaner and he should pause and listen to them when they begin.

By 4 Months
He should quieten or smile to the sound of your voice even when he cannot see you. He may also turn his head or eyes toward you if you come up from behind and speak to him from the side.

By 7 Months
He should turn immediately to your voice across the room or to very quiet noises made on each side if he is not too occupied with other things.

By 9 Months
He should listen attentively to familiar everyday sounds and search for very quiet sounds made out of sight. He should also show pleasure in babbling loudly and tunefully.

By 12 Months
He should show some response to his own name and to other familiar words. He may also respond when you say 'no' and 'bye bye' even when he cannot see any accompanying gesture.

> Your health visitor will perform a routine hearing screening test on your baby between six and eight months of age. She will be able to help and advise you at any time before or after this test if you are concerned about your baby and his development. If you suspect that your baby is not hearing normally, either because you cannot answer yes to the items above or for some other reason, then seek advice from your health visitor.

©
Produced by Dr. Barry McCormick
Children's Hearing Assessment Centre, General Hospital, Nottingham NG1 6HA
Printed by The Sherwood Press (Nottingham) Limited

Figure 1.3. The author's 'Can your baby hear you?' checklist is used widely in the UK.

detected following referrals from the Health Visitors' Distraction test and the test achieved high coverage (96%) and had a sensitivity of 88%.

Targeted neonatal hearing screening has the potential to catch 40% of congenitally deaf babies if performed on the special care baby group (roughly 7% of births) and if well babies with family history of child-hood deafness and others with known relevant syndromes are also included. Tests utilising auditory brainstem responses (ABR) and oto-acoustic emissions (OAE) have been favoured in recent years although other 'behavioural' methods have also been developed, including an Auditory Response Cradle (Tucker and Bhattacharya, 1992). Mass screening at the neonatal stage has the potential to catch 70% of deaf babies and the ones that will not be detected include those with progressive or acquired losses, the false negatives from the tests, and those discharged prior to testing. Community hearing screening and surveillance will be needed to detect the 30–60% of babies not detected by neonatal screens or all cases in the absence of neonatal tests.

Infants beyond the first year of life and into the school years will require the screening and observation methods detailed in this book. The intention should be to ensure that all cases with hearing losses in excess of 40 dB are provided with hearing aids, cochlear implants or manual communication and all cases with lesser degrees of hearing loss are monitored carefully and given appropriate treatment where indicated.

Failure to acknowledge the presence of a hearing problem in childhood and failure to arrange appropriate investigation and support must be considered to fall into the category of negligence. The time has never been more opportune for the medical practitioner to be informed of what can be done and what should be done to detect and to support hearing-impaired children. Knowledge of the investigations, the procedures, the terminology and of how to interpret results will be found within the following pages.

References

Davis, A. C. and Sancho, J. (1988). Screening for hearing impairment in children: a review of current UK practice with special reference to the screening of babies from Special Care Baby Units for severe/profound hearing impairment. In *Human Communication Disorders: A Worldwide Perspective* (ed. S. Gerber), pp. 237–75. Washington: Galaudet.

Davis, A. C. and Wood, S. (1992). The epidemiology of childhood hearing impairment: factors relevant to planning of services. *British Journal of Audiology*, **26**, 77–90.

McCormick, B. (1983). Hearing screening by health visitors: a critical appraisal of the distraction test. *Health Visitor*, **56**, 449–51.

McCormick, B. (1991). *Screening for Hearing Impairment in Young Children*. London: Chapman & Hall.

National Institutes of Health (1993). NIH Consensus Statement: Early Identification of Hearing Impairment in Infants and Young Children, Vol. 11, Number 1.

Tucker, S. M. and Bhattacharya, J. (1992). Screening of hearing impairment in the newborn using the auditory response cradle. *Archives of Disease in Childhood*, **67**, 911–19.

2

Causes of deafness

KEVIN P. GIBBIN

Causes of deafness

In considering a topic as wide ranging as deafness it is important to
have a framework on which to hang the main elements to be discussed.
There are many different ways of classifying deafness, two of which will
be used for this chapter. With the framework established, salient points
within each category will be discussed.

The most fundamental classification system is based on the site of the
hearing loss and therefore on the nature of the loss. Deafness may
result from pathology in the external or middle-ear causing a conductive hearing loss – a failure of transmission of the sound signal from the
outside world to the inner ear. Sensorineural deafness arises from
pathology either within the inner ear, a sensory or cochlear loss, or
from pathology in the neural pathways connecting with the brain, a
neural or retrocochlear deafness. With the development of cochlear
implantation as a means of treating profound deafness it is no longer
only of academic interest to differentiate between these two groups of
causes of deafness; cochlear implantation is of benefit only if the central
neural pathways remain intact and is therefore not appropriate in cases
of retrocochlear deafness. Conductive deafness is considerably more
common than sensorineural deafness, the latter having a prevalence of
one or two per thousand (Davis and Wood, 1992).

In addition to the two main sub-groups, conductive and sensorineural
deafness, a third extremely rare group may be identified, central deafness, in which the pathology lies within the auditory cortex. It is also
important to remember that even in childhood, typically in older children, non-organic deafness may be seen. Conductive deafness usually
produces either a low tone or a relatively flat hearing loss with all

frequencies being equally affected. The maximum degree of deafness from a conductive loss is about 60 dB. Sensorineural deafness varies from a very minor loss to a total loss of hearing with varying auditory patterns on the pure tone audiogram, a high frequency deafness being a common finding.

The second system of classification to be used here is based upon when the deafness occurs and whether or not there is a genetic element to the aetiology. The system may be outlined:

Prenatal causes
Perinatal causes
Postnatal causes

There may be a genetic element in both prenatal and postnatal causes of deafness and of course the nature of the loss may be conductive or sensorineural. In addition it should be noted that deafness may occur in a variety of syndromes; in some it is an essential element of the syndrome, in others it is an optional inclusion. Hearing loss as part of a syndrome may be present from birth or it may occur at a later stage.

Prenatal causes

Of the non-genetic prenatal causes of deafness two major factors have been eliminated over the past 20 years or so. Rhesus haemolytic disease and associated kernicterus is now a rare cause of neonatal deafness thanks to the development of anti-D inoculation in cases of maternofoetal rhesus incompatibility. Similarly rubella as a cause of morbidity, including deafness, has to all intents and purposes been eliminated due to rubella immunisation of young girls.

Maternal infection during pregnancy may result in materno-foetal transmission of the infecting agent; rubella as a cause of deafness has already been referred to but other infections are still a significant cause of morbidity. Cytomegalovirus (CMV) is a cause of congenital sensorineural deafness; this may be associated with severe handicap if the infection is obvious at birth. In subclinical cases the prognosis is often better. Culture of the virus may be obtained from urine in the first few weeks of life. Serology will confirm the diagnosis, showing a rising titre of IgG antibody or the presence of CMV-specific IgM. Toxoplasmosis, caused by *Toxoplasma gondii*, is another cause of congenital sensorineural deafness; serum antibody titres will help make the diagnosis.

Drugs are now used with much greater caution in pregnancy and disasters such as occurred with thalidomide are much less likely as a result. Non-genetic developmental abnormalities of the ears may however still occur as a result of random mutation or chance effects on the developing foetus. These effects may be on the inner ear during its development from otic placode, a neuro-ectodermal derivative, or on the middle and external ears; the former develops from the tubotympanic recess, an out-pouching of the first pharyngeal pouch, the latter from the first visceral cleft. All these events take place between the fifth and fourteenth week of gestation. Developmental abnormalities may be grouped in four separate categories:

> abnormalities of the pinna; these range from minor cosmetic abnormalities to total aplasia
> abnormalities of the external auditory canal including total aplasia
> abnormalities of the middle-ear cleft, including ossicular abnormalities
> abnormalities of the inner ear and central auditory pathways

Developmental anomalies of the inner ear are rare and include such conditions as Mondini dysplasia in which the cochlea develops as a single coil.

Genetic abnormalities may result in any of the above abnormalities and many well defined deafness syndromes exist; however deafness may be an isolated feature, due either to dominant autosomal transmission or to a recessive inheritance. In the latter case the diagnosis will be made by a process of exclusion. Deafness syndromes may have a genetic basis although many do not. Various classification systems exist; one convenient classification groups the auditory defect with defects in other systems or parts of the body:

Deafness associated with:

> skeletal/craniofacial abnormalities – examples include Apert's syndrome (acrocephalosyndactyly), Crouzon's syndrome, Klippel–Fiel syndrome, cleft palate and lip and Treacher–Collin's syndrome;
> neurological disorders – a typical example is cerebral palsy;
> epidermal/pigmentary disorders – Waardenburg's syndrome is a well known example in which there are white areas of hair in the forelock, eyebrows and eyelashes and heterochromia iridis;

ophthalmological disorders – Usher's syndrome – deafness associated with retinitis pigmentosa;

metabolic/endocrine/renal disorders – Alport's syndrome (deafness and progressive hereditary nephritis) and Pendred's syndrome (deafness associated with goitre) are examples;

chromosomal abnormalities – Down's syndrome, Turner's syndrome, trisomy 13–15 and trisomy 18 are examples;

other miscellaneous conditions – examples include CHARGE syndrome (Coloboma, Heart disease, Atretic posterior nasal choanae, Retarded development, Genital hypoplasia and Ear anomalies).

Perinatal causes

With increasing success by obstetricians and paediatricians in resuscitating very low birth weight preterm infants has come the awareness that many of these children have a much higher incidence than their normal birth weight/full term peers of suffering from sensorineural deafness (Davis and Wood, 1992). Low birth weight may be associated with a variety of factors including traumatic delivery, neonatal asphyxia and hypoxia and respiratory distress syndrome. Neonatal acidosis may also contribute as may intracranial haemorrhage. It has also been suggested that the neonatal cochlea may be unduly susceptible to noise, concern being raised about incubator noise.

Postnatal causes

Postnatal causes of deafness can mean either a conductive or a sensorineural loss. Sensorineural loss may develop from genetic causes, both dominant and recessive, either as an isolated lesion or as part of a syndrome with the deafness as a late onset feature. Children with progressive sensorineural deafness are encountered and prove to be a particularly difficult group to manage due to doubt about the possibility of overlooking a treatable lesion such as a labyrinthine fistula.

Non-genetic causes of acquired sensorineural deafness include meningitis, mumps (in which the loss is typically unilateral), measles, trauma and, rarely, exposure to ototoxic agents. Meningitis remains the commonest cause of acquired sensorineural deafness in childhood (Martin, 1982), the pathology being a septic labyrinthitis as a result of spread of infection from the cerebrospinal fluid to the perilymph through the cochlear aqueduct. Any one of three major infecting agents causing meningitis, *Haemophilus influenzae*, *Neisseria meningitidis* and *Streptococcus pneumoniae*, may cause deafness; although much more rare, tuberculous meningitis is associated with a high incidence of hearing loss.

Conductive deafness

Rarely conductive deafness may be congenital, as for example in the Treacher–Collin's syndrome in which there may be total atresia of the pinna and external auditory canals. However the commonest causes of conductive deafness are acquired due to inflammatory conditions of the external auditory meatus or middle ear.

Conductive losses account for the greatest number of children with deafness, with otitis media with effusion (OME) being the single most common cause. It must be remembered that children with sensorineural deafness are not precluded from developing a conductive loss due to OME and this must not be overlooked in the diagnosis and treatment of deaf children. Indeed it is particularly important that an acquired conductive deafness due to OME in a child with a severe or profound hearing loss should be detected as soon as possible.

Many causes of conductive deafness produce a short term impairment, often unilateral, as in cases of acute suppurative otitis media (ASOM). ASOM affects large numbers of children, 84% experiencing this at some stage in early life.

Chronic suppurative otitis media (CSOM) is considerably less common; it is considered under two broad headings, tubotympanic disease and attico-antral disease. Tubotympanic disease is the more common of the two; the underlying pathology is a chronic mucositis of the middle-ear, characterised clinically by a central tympanic perforation with mucopurulent discharge. The underlying mucositis may resolve and the tympanic membrane may heal with no residual deficit, either in the hearing or on otoscopy. However in some cases the eardrum may fail to heal leaving a dry perforation of the pars tensa. The effects of such disease on the hearing depend on the size and location of the perforation and on any effects on the ossicular chain. A small anterior perforation may produce no hearing loss at all and conversely a large posterior perforation may produce a moderate conductive loss.

Attico-antral disease is often associated with a normal mesotympanum, the disease, as the name implies, being confined to the attic with a pars flaccida defect and associated with cholesteatoma; discharge may be very scanty and is usually offensive. The hearing loss in these cases will depend on the nature of any damage to the ossicular chain; there may be erosion of the tip of the long process of the incus producing an ossicular discontinuity and a conductive loss of up to 60 dB, the maximum possible loss for a purely conductive deafness. Fortunately most cases of attico-antral disease are unilateral.

Otitis media with effusion (OME), as already noted, is the single commonest cause of deafness in childhood with a prevalence varying from 7 to 19% (Tos *et al.*, 1986). OME occurs throughout early childhood; Birch and Elbrond (1984) have shown that the maximum proportion of children with tympanometric evidence of effusions was found in 1-year-olds. There is a marked seasonal variation in the incidence of OME; Rach, Zeilhuis and van den Broek (1986) demonstrated that 39% of ears had tympanometric evidence of OME in winter compared with 24% in summer. Gibb (1979) has stated that malfunction of the Eustachian tube is the essential underlying cause of OME, but this is to oversimplify matters. Clearly Eustachian dysfunction does play a role in the aetiology of OME, as shown for example in the high incidence of OME in children with cleft palate. Other factors to be considered include the role of the adenoids, whether it be due to the adenoid mass obstructing the tubal opening in the nasopharynx, infection in the adenoids or their histamine content. It is generally agreed that OME is a truly multifactorial condition with tubal function and anatomy as perhaps the more important elements, with infection and mucosal factors also playing a part.

The hearing loss in OME varies. Sade (1979) demonstrated an average loss of 28 dB, but the auditory threshold may fluctuate despite persistence of the effusion. The deafness in OME may present in a variety of ways, in some instances determined by the age of the child. The loss may be detected on routine screening of hearing at the 9 month stage and Haggard *et al.* (1992) have shown an incidence of referrable (to an otolaryngologist) severity of middle-ear disease of 1.3% of the age cohort. The deafness may present as failure to develop normal patterns of speech and language and in this context it has been suggested that the fluctuating nature of the loss in OME may be more damaging than a more severe persistent loss as may be seen in sensorineural deafness. Hall and Hill (1986) have considered five factors in assessing why OME can have a major effect in some children and yet be trivial in others:

1. the age at which the disorders occur
2. the duration of the episodes
3. the severity of the loss
4. intrinsic qualities in the child
5. the child's environment

Children with OME may present with behaviour disturbances and in older, school age, children the hearing loss may present as underachievement in class, particularly in reading skills. In a small number of children there may be long term sequelae as a result of OME, with collapse of the tympanic membrane (atelectasis), adhesive otitis and tympanosclerosis. These sequelae may be associated with a permanent conductive loss.

Other causes of conductive loss in children are uncommon. Other than foreign bodies in the external auditory meatus, acute conditions of the ear canal are uncommon. Trauma – head injury – may cause disruption of the ossicular chain, as may unskilled attempts at removal of foreign bodies. Other possible effects of trauma include haemotympanum, blood in the middle ear, which usually resolves completely; it is, however, possible for adhesions to develop after bleeding into the middle ear and a persistent conductive loss to occur. A perforation may also be caused by trauma.

References

Birch, L. and Elbrond, O. (1984). Prospective epidemiological investigation of secretory otitis media in children attending day care centres. *ORL*, **46**, 229–34.

Davis, A. and Wood, S. (1992). The epidemiology of childhood hearing impairment: factors relevant to planning of services. *British Journal of Audiology*, **25**, 77–90.

Gibb, A. G. (1979). Non-suppurative otitis media. In *Scott-Brown's Diseases of the Ear, Nose and Throat*, 4th edn (ed. J. Ballantyne and J. Groves), pp. 193–236, London: Butterworths.

Haggard, M. P., McCormick, B., Gannon, M. M. and Spencer, H. (1992). The paediatric otological caseload resulting from improved screening in the first year of life. *Clinical Otolaryngology*, **17**, 34–43.

Hall, D. M. B. and Hill, P. (1986). When does secretory otitis media affect language development? *Archives of Disease in Childhood*, **61**, 42–7.

Martin, J. A. M. (1982). Aetiological factors relating to childhood deafness in the European Community. *Audiology*, **21**, 149–58.

Rach, G. H., Zeilhuis, G. A. and van den Broek, P. (1986). The prevalence of otitis media with effusion in two year old children in the Netherlands. In *Acute and Secretory Otitis* (ed. J. Sade), pp. 136–7. Amsterdam: Kugler.

Sade, J. (1979). *Secretory Otitis Media and its Sequelae*. New York: Churchill Livingstone.
Tos, M., Stangerup, S. E., Hvid, G., Andreassen, U. K. and Thomsen, J. (1986). Epidemiology and natural history of secretory otitis. In *Acute and Secretory Otitis* (ed. J. Sade), pp. 95–106. Amsterdam: Kugler.

3

Behavioural tests

ANGELA MAXWELL

Behavioural hearing tests require the child to show an overt response to an auditory stimulus. The response may be a head turn or a play response such as putting a peg in a board. These tests give important information about the child's ability to detect and process sound, unlike objective techniques, which investigate different parts of the auditory pathway. For this reason, results from objective hearing tests should always be interpreted in the light of behavioural findings, to give an overall picture of how a child responds to sound.

The aim of paediatric behavioural testing is to determine, as accurately and reliably as possible, the presence and nature of any hearing impairment and the threshold of hearing across the important speech frequency range, from 500 Hz up to 4 kHz. The choice of test technique is based on the developmental age of the child, not necessarily the chronological age. Table 3.1 outlines the different test techniques and their ages for application. Behavioural audiological tests should always be accompanied by impedance measurements to investigate the status of the middle ear and the integrity of the acoustic reflex arc. (See Chapter 6 for further details of impedance measurements.)

Behavioural testing of children's hearing can be divided into the two separate but overlapping areas of auditory detection and auditory discrimination. Techniques involving auditory detection can be used from the age of a few weeks. As the child matures, so the response develops, from a reflex involuntary change in behaviour, for example arousal from sleep, to a voluntary conditioned response, where the child must wait and then carry out a simple action, on hearing an auditory stimulus. Auditory discrimination tasks cannot be incorporated into the audiological assessment until a child is 18–24 months developmentally, at which time he or she should be able to carry out simple verbal

Table 3.1 *Choice of test technique and developmental age*

Developmental age (months)	Choice of test technique	
	Auditory detection	Auditory discrimination
0–6	Behavioural observation audiometry	–
6–18	Distraction test VRA	–
18–30	Distraction test VRA	Cooperative test
30–60	VRA Performance test Pure tone audiometry	Speech discrimination tests, e.g. the McCormick Toy Discrimination Test, the Kendall Toy Test

instructions. Beyond this age assessment should involve measures of the child's auditory detection and auditory discrimination skills. This chapter aims to give a brief explanation of screening and diagnostic paediatric hearing tests used throughout the UK. A more comprehensive account can be found in *Paediatric Audiology 0–5 Years*, edited by McCormick (1993).

Auditory detection

1. Behavioural observation audiometry

Up to the age of 6 months, it is difficult to implement any formal test technique to obtain information regarding hearing thresholds. However, skilled observation by an experienced tester of a baby's consistent change in behaviour, for example eye widening or a startle in response to auditory stimulation, can give reliable information about a baby's hearing sensitivity. In this age group, for normally hearing babies, responses can be elicited only to moderate–intensely raised levels, not at threshold levels. More objective methods such as otoacoustic emission investigations (see Chapter 5) and impedance measurements can provide additional information about middle- and inner-ear function. Depending on the findings from both behavioural and objective measurements, the audiologist may decide to review the baby when he is developmentally ready for full distraction testing or to refer him for auditory brainstem response (ABR) investigations. Mason, McCormick and Wood (1988) have found that in Nottingham only 3% of children seen for behavioural audiological assessment need to be referred on for ABR measurements.

2. The Distraction Test

By 6–7 months of age, most babies are sufficiently mature to sit unsupported and are able to turn to locate quiet sounds presented out of vision and level with the ear, if they are not too engrossed in other activities. This is the principle on which the Distraction Test is based and it was first described by Ewing and Ewing in 1944. It is widely used by health visitors in the community as a screening test for babies aged 6–7 months, as well as being used diagnostically in audiological clinics.

The Distraction Test is a sensitive and reliable test for detecting hearing loss in this age group, if administered by skilled, well-trained testers (McCormick, 1988). However, there are a number of pitfalls that testers must be aware of to ensure that the technique is assessing only hearing sensitivity and not other sensory functions. Such pitfalls include allowing the sound source, or tester, to enter the baby's peripheral visual field, resulting in visual cueing, and using broadband auditory stimuli instead of frequency specific stimuli to assess the hearing sensitivity. For a comprehensive discussion including such sources of error, the reader is referred to *Screening for Hearing Impairment in Young Children*, by McCormick (1988).

Test procedure

The Distraction Test requires the baby to be seated erect on the mother's lap and two trained testers, one located in front of the baby, and one located out of vision behind the baby. The front tester captures, controls and phases the baby's attention using simple toys on a low table. As the distracter phases the baby's attention, the second tester presents the auditory stimulus out of view, level with the baby's ear (see Figure 3.1). A baby with normal hearing should respond by turning to locate the stimulus (see Figure 3.2).

The test aims to assess a child's hearing sensitivity to low, mid and high frequencies bilaterally, using frequency-specific stimuli (see Table 3.2). The use of sounds with a broadband frequency spectrum, for example, tissue paper or whispered and voiced speech, are not suitable for such assessment. During the screening distraction test, each stimulus must be presented at a level determined by each health authority, and this should be in the region of 35 dB(A).

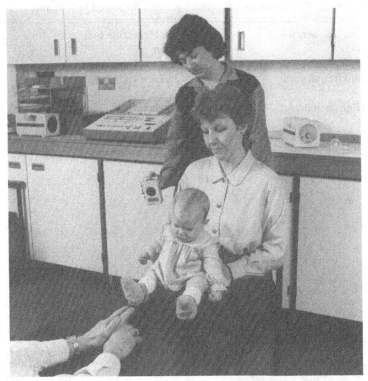

Figure 3.1. The Distraction Test demonstrating presentation of the auditory stimulus.

Pass criteria

To pass the screening test, the baby must make a full head turn to locate each stimulus presented at the screening level, for example 35 dB(A). The baby must respond reliably to two out of three presentations, to low, mid and high frequency stimuli on each side. If a baby consistently fails to respond to any of the sounds, then he or she fails the screen and a follow-up hearing assessment should be arranged, either a second screen or further diagnostic testing.

Reasons for failure

A failed hearing screen can result from many factors, not necessarily related to poor hearing sensitivity. It may be that the baby is not yet developmentally ready for the test if not sitting unsupported or has poor head control. Alternatively, the baby's attention state may not be optimal on the day of testing. A baby's responsiveness to tactile and

Table 3.2 *Frequency-specific stimuli suitable for sound field testing*

Low frequencies	500 Hz warble tone Hum
Mid frequencies	2 kHz warble tone
High frequencies	4 kHz warble tone Manchester rattle 's' consonant

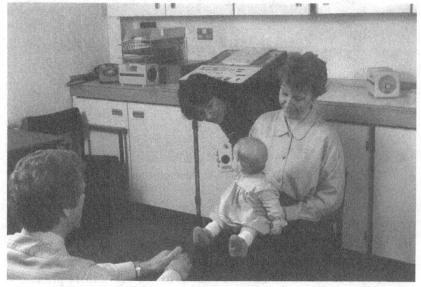

Figure 3.2. The head turn response to locate the auditory stimulus.

visual stimulation during distraction testing can give important clues to the child's attention state. If a baby is quick to such stimuli, but shows a consistent lack of awareness to auditory stimuli, then the presence of a hearing impairment is strongly indicated.

One of the most common reasons for failing a hearing screen is middle-ear dysfunction, typically otitis media with effusion (OME). This can cause a temporary, but in some cases persistent, mild–moderate loss of hearing sensitivity. The presence of middle-ear fluid does not automatically indicate a significant loss of hearing sensitivity and this is one

Table 3.3 *Degree of hearing loss related to response level*

Hearing sensitivity	Response level (dB(A))
Normal	<35
Mild	35–40
Moderate	41–70
Severe	71–95
Profound	>95

of the reasons why impedance measurements are too sensitive for screening programmes. Any failed hearing test should be taken seriously and further assessment must be arranged.

Diagnostic distraction techniques adhere to the same basic principles as the screening test, but the levels at which the stimuli are presented differ. The aim of the test is to record the quietest level at which the baby responds, using a range of stimuli covering the speech frequency range, from 500 Hz up to 4 kHz. The stimuli are raised from quiet levels below 35 dB(A) until the baby turns to locate two out of three presentations at consistent levels for each sound. The degree of any hearing impairment is categorised depending on the response levels recorded and averaged over the frequency range 500–4000 Hz (see Table 3.3).

The presence of otitis media can lead to reduced hearing up to a moderate level of approximately 65 dB(A). Levels greater than this may indicate the presence of a sensorineural or mixed loss, that is, an underlying sensorineural hearing loss. If a baby presents with consistently raised levels on distraction testing, in the absence of any conductive element, there is a strong indication of a sensorineural hearing impairment and amplification may be required.

3. Visual reinforcement audiometry

Visual reinforcement audiometry (VRA) is a powerful and reliable technique that can be used to assess the hearing sensitivity in the age group 6–9 months, up to about 3 years of age. It is a technique used less widely in the UK than in America and Australia, particularly at a screening level, mainly because the equipment needed is not easily portable. It can, however, be particularly useful for difficult-to-test children or those with additional handicaps.

Test procedure

The essence of VRA is to visually reward and reinforce a particular behaviour, which is generally a head turn to locate a frequency-specific sound. On turning to locate the sound source, the child receives a visual reward, for example flashing lights on a soft toy. The clear reward, associated with locating the sound, may hold the child's attention better than the Distraction Test (Moore, Thompson and Thompson, 1975) and is particularly useful for those babies who are too mature for distraction testing. For a more detailed discussion of VRA, the reader is referred to Bamford and McSporran, Chapter 5 in *Paediatric Audiology 0–5 Years*, edited by McCormick (1993).

Most diagnostic clinics using VRA require two testers to be involved. The first is outside the test room, controlling the presentation of the auditory stimuli from a remote audiometer whilst observing through a one-way observation window. The second tester remains in the room with the parent and child and controls the child's attention. In cases involving shy and withdrawn children, the second tester can leave the room and observe the child's responses through the window. In practice, this method often increases the test time, but can mean the difference between obtaining important audiological data and obtaining little, if any, information about the child's hearing sensitivity.

The aim of VRA, as with distraction testing, is to record the quietest level at which the child consistently responds to frequency-specific stimuli, typically 500 Hz, 2 kHz and 4 kHz warble tones. Initially, the visual reward and the auditory stimulus, presented at a suprathreshold level, are paired to condition the child to turn to one side. The auditory stimulus is then presented alone and the visual reward activated only when the child has turned to locate the sound source (Figure 3.3). The stimulus level is then lowered and raised until the quietest level needed to initiate a response is found.

As the response is a conditioned response, many centres tend to test on one side only. The child's localisation abilities can be observed at the start of the test, when presenting the initial auditory stimulus. It is necessary to explain clearly to the parents that the technique assesses essentially the ear with the better hearing and in doing so, the child's overall hearing sensitivity.

Typically, VRA is used to assess a child's hearing in the sound field.

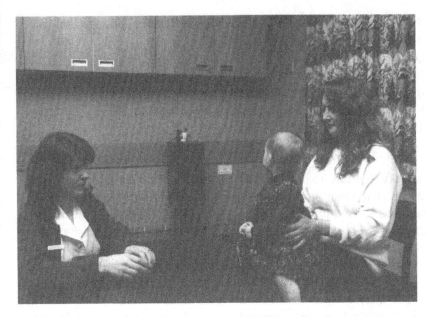

Figure 3.3. Visual reinforcement audiometry demonstrating the head turn response and visual reward.

Some centres now routinely use VRA with insert earphones or headphones, to obtain ear-specific results (Borton *et al.*, 1989). Gravel and Traquina (1992) found that they could obtain frequency-specific data during the initial assessment session, either under headphones or in the sound field, from 90% of infants aged 6–24 months. Ear-specific results were recorded in 84% of cases. They concluded that VRA can provide ear- and frequency-specific estimates of hearing thresholds in young infants.

VRA can also be undertaken using bone conduction measurements, to investigate the presence of a sensorineural impairment or an air–bone gap, consistent with a conductive component (Horner and Horner, 1979). See Chapter 4 for further details on bone conduction measurements and results.

4. The Performance Test

By the developmental age of 2½ years onwards, most children can be conditioned to wait for an auditory stimulus and then carry out a particular action, for example, putting a peg in a board. This is the basic principle of the Performance Test. The great advantage of this test is that the child can be conditioned through demonstration only – no language is required. This has obvious implications for those children with language delays or disorders and for those whose first language is not English. The aim of the Performance Test is to record the quietest level the child consistently responds to bilaterally, using frequency-specific stimuli across the speech frequency range, typically 500 Hz, 2 kHz and 4 kHz.

Test procedures

Initially, the task required is demonstrated several times by the tester, using clear visual and suprathreshold auditory stimuli. The auditory stimulus is then presented, without the visual cues, at 45° behind the child, at ear level on one side (Figure 3.4). The stimulus intensity is lowered to a minimal level, for example 35 dB(A), and raised if the child does not respond, until a consistent threshold is obtained for each frequency on both sides.

The Performance Test is often used as a screening technique by health visitors in the community. In this situation, the child must respond to two out of three presentations at each frequency bilaterally, at the agreed screening intensity level (for example 35 dB(A)) to pass the screen.

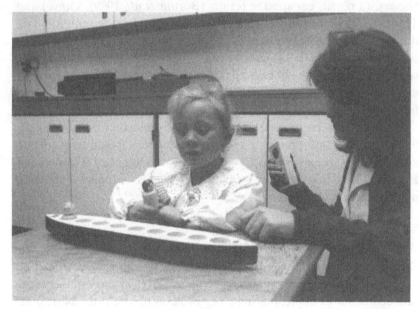

Figure 3.4. The Performance Test.

Once a child can be conditioned reliably, then in theory he is ready for pure tone audiometry (see Chapter 4). However, one obstacle to obtaining such ear-specific measurements is the child's reluctance to accept headphones. This is a common occurrence in children below the age of 3 years. In some cases, it may be possible to persuade the child to wear the bone vibrator, enabling the tester to obtain bone-conduction measurements to investigate inner-ear function.

Auditory discrimination

From the developmental age of 18 months onwards, most children are able to understand and carry out simple verbal instructions. However, this age group is often the most difficult and challenging to assess, because of general lack of cooperation in adult-controlled activities. The skills of fully trained and experienced testers (with an abundance of patience) are required to obtain reliable and accurate results. It must be remembered that speech discrimination tests cannot be used solely as a test of a child's hearing sensitivity. Such methods must be accompanied by age-appropriate auditory detection tests to assess the child's hearing at specific frequencies across the speech frequency range.

1. The Cooperative Test

The principles behind this technique are to develop a 'giving' game with the child, using simple instructions and familiar words. The test is more sensitive if acoustically similar words are used: for example, teddy, dolly, baby, mummy, daddy.

Test procedure

The 'game' is established by demonstrating the activity, and saying 'give it to mummy/baby/teddy', initially with visual cues and using a loud conversational voice level. The child is then encouraged to participate in the 'game'. The tester should cover his or her mouth to eliminate visual cues and reduce the voice to a level of less than 40 dB(A) without whispering. The tester must ensure that quiet, voiced speech is used because whispering can cause distortion of the sound signal leading to inaccurate results (Figure 3.5).

The aim is to record the quietest listening level needed for the child to score 80%, that is to carry out four out of five instructions correctly, without the aid of lipreading. Children with normal hearing sensitivity

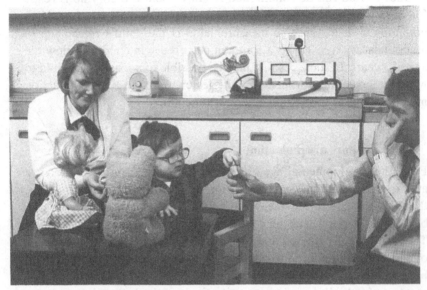

Figure 3.5. The Cooperative Test.

and who are developmentally ready for the test, can complete the task at listening levels of less than 40 dB(A).

2. Speech discrimination tests

From 18 months onwards, a child's vocabulary and language increases dramatically. By the age of 2–2½ years, most children are able to participate in speech discrimination tasks using specific speech material, for example the Kendall Toy Test (Kendall, 1954) and the Toy Discrimination Test (McCormick, 1977).

Speech tasks for use with this age group must be simple, quick and specifically designed with young children in mind. In 1977, McCormick designed the Toy Discrimination Test to meet these criteria and to be used as a screening test by health visitors in the community. When applied to children, some as young as 2 years of age, the test establishes the quietest voice level at which the child can reliably discriminate between acoustically similar speech sounds. The test consists of simple, familiar items, for example, a shoe and a cup, rather than pictures, as real objects tend to hold young children's interest more and are less abstract.

Test procedure

The Toy Discrimination Test consists of seven paired items, for example, cup/duck, shoe/spoon which, when displayed on a low table, are used in a finger-pointing game. Not all the pairs need to be used to ensure a high level of sensitivity. With young children especially, only two or three pairs may be used.

The tester, using a normal conversational voice level, asks the child to find several items using the simple phrase, 'give me the ...' or 'show me the ...'. Once the 'game' is established, the tester covers the mouth and reduces his or her voice level to a minimal level of 40 dB(A) (Figure 3.6). To pass this screening test in the community, the child must correctly identify four out of five items on request at 40 dB(A), without lipreading.

The Toy Discrimination Test is also used widely in audiology clinics in the UK as a diagnostic tool. If the child is unable to identify the items at less than 40 dB(A), the voice level is raised and lowered, to determine the quietest level at which the child obtains an 80% success rate.

One of the obvious problems associated with speech discrimination tasks using live voice, is that of intra- and inter-subject variability. There can be problems with maintaining the voice at minimal levels and

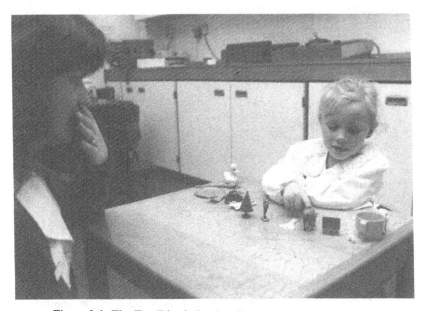

Figure 3.6. The Toy Discrimination Test.

of distorting the speech signal. To overcome these and other sources of error, McCormick, in conjunction with colleagues from the Medical Research Council's Institute of Hearing Research, devised an automated version of the Toy Discrimination Test, known as the IHR/McCormick Automated Toy Discrimination Test (Figure 3.7). The idea of using digital recording of speech for application in this test came from Professor Mark Haggard.

The lead-in phrases and toy items were recorded by a female speaker and are reproduced automatically through a loudspeaker, by pressing the appropriate button on a handset. In this way, the problems of controlling voice levels are overcome and greater accuracy is obtained because lower voice levels can be used than can be produced consistently via live voice presentation. The level the words are presented at is lowered and raised, depending on whether the child's response is right or wrong, until five reversals have occurred. The handset then displays the speech discrimination threshold giving a 71% correct response. This automated version has proved to be accurate and reliable and allows greater sensitivity than when using live voice presentation (Ousey *et al.*, 1989)

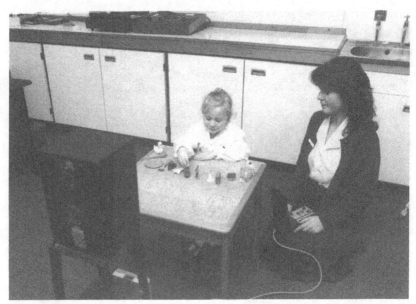

Figure 3.7. The IHR/McCormick Automated Toy Discrimination Test.

Further investigations using the automated Toy Discrimination Test have demonstrated that the speech discrimination score obtained can be used as a basis for estimating the puretone thresholds at 500 Hz, 1 kHz and 4 kHz, in the child's better ear (Palmer, Sheppard and Marshall, 1991). The correlation was found to be high with a 95% confidence interval of 11 dB. This version of the Toy Discrimination Test is not and cannot be fully automated. The tester still needs experience and skill in handling young children and controlling their attention, so that reliable and accurate results are obtained.

Summary

Children of all ages can undergo audiological assessment using behavioural methods. The choice of test technique depends on the developmental age of the child, not the chronological age. The testing of young children can be a difficult and challenging task, requiring experience and skill in child handling and interaction, interpretation of test results and parental counselling. Therefore, hearing assessment must be carried out by fully trained and competent testers. Early detection and appropriate early intervention for hearing impaired children is paramount. Studies have shown that amplification at an early age can lead to improved speech and language skills, as well as having important implications for social and emotional development.

References

Bamford, J. and McSporran, E. (1993). Visual reinforcement audiometry. In *Paediatric Audiology 0–5 years*, 2nd cdn, ed. B. McCormick, pp. 124–55. London: Whurr Publishers Limited.

Borton, T. E., Nolen, B. L., Luks, S. B. and Meline, N. C. (1989). Clinical applicability of insert earphones for audiometry. *Audiology*, **28**, 61–70.

Ewing, I. R. and Ewing, A. W. G. (1944). The ascertainment of deafness in infancy and early childhood. *Journal of Laryngology and Otology*, **59**, 309–38.

Gravel, J. S. and Traquina, D. N. (1992). Experience with the audiological assessment of infants and toddlers. *International Journal of Pediatric Otorhinolaryngology*, **23**, 59–71.

Horner, J. S. and Horner, J. P. (1979). Puretone earphone and BC thresholds on 5–11 month infants. *Proceedings of American Speech and Hearing Association*, Atlanta, USA.

Kendall, D. C. (1954). Audiometry for young children. *Teacher of the Deaf*, **307**, 18–23.

Mason, S., McCormick, B. and Wood, S. (1988). Auditory brainstem response in paediatric audiology. *Archives of Disease in Childhood*, **64**, 465–7.

McCormick, B. (1977). The Toy Discrimination Test: an aid for screening the hearing of children above a mental age of 2 years. *Public Health*, **91**, 67–73.

McCormick, B. (1988). *Screening for Hearing Impairment in Young Children*. London: Chapman & Hall.

McCormick, B. (ed.) (1993). *Paediatric Audiology 0–5 Years*, 2nd edn. London: Whurr Publishers Limited.

Moore, J. M., Thompson, G. and Thompson, M. (1975). Auditory localisation of infants as a function of reinforcement conditions. *Journal of Speech and Hearing Disorders*, **40**, 29–34.

Ousey, J., Sheppard, S., Twomey, T. and Palmer, A. R. (1989). The IHR/McCormick Automated Toy Discrimination Test – description and initial evaluation. *British Journal of Audiology*, **23**, 245–51.

Palmer, A. R., Sheppard, S. and Marshall, D. H. (1991). Prediction of hearing thresholds in children using an automated toy discrimination test. *British Journal of Audiology*, **25**, 351–6.

4

Pure tone audiometry

SALLY WOOD

Introduction

Pure tone audiometry is the most commonly used procedure for the measurement of hearing loss in older children and adults. Pure tone signals (i.e. tones with a single frequency of vibration) are delivered to the patient via headphones or a bone vibrator. The patient's threshold of hearing at each frequency of interest is measured using a standard technique and the thresholds compared with normal values in order to quantify the degree of hearing loss. In addition comparison of air-conduction and bone-conduction thresholds (the air–bone gap) can often give useful information about the type of hearing loss.

This chapter describes the equipment and techniques used to obtain pure tone audiograms with particular reference to the modifications necessary for paediatric work. It also describes the interpretation of audiograms and the limitations of the technique.

The audiometer

Audiometers range from simple screening instruments with a limited range of test frequencies and intensities to complex diagnostic instruments with facilities for a wide range of clinical tests in addition to threshold measurement. Signals may be presented via headphones (air conduction) or via a bone vibrator (bone conduction).

Frequency

The frequencies of interest are in the range 125 to 8000 Hz at octave intervals (an octave corresponds to a doubling of the frequency range), i.e.

125, 250, 500, 1000, 2000, 4000, 8000 Hz

The following intermediate frequencies may also be of interest:

750, 1500, 3000, 6000

Typically, in paediatric work, thresholds would be obtained for the frequency range 500–4000 Hz and other frequencies tested as necessary.

Intensity

The intensity is usually calibrated in 5 dB steps and typically extends from –10 dB up to a maximum value that varies with frequency but is usually around 120 dB for air-conduction stimuli in the mid frequencies. For bone-conduction stimuli the maximum output available is usually considerably lower, at around the 60–80 dB level depending upon the particular audiometer.

The dBHL scale has been designed specifically for measurements obtained with pure tone audiometers and is constructed such that 0 dBHL at each frequency corresponds to the normal threshold of hearing at that frequency. The actual acoustical output in terms of sound pressure level required to reach threshold is different at each frequency as the human ear is not uniformly sensitive across the frequency range. It would be cumbersome and inconvenient to have a different normal reference level at each frequency and the dBHL scale was devised to overcome this requirement. When a patient's hearing threshold is reported in dBHL for a given frequency, this is a statement of how much better or worse their hearing is at that frequency than the internationally accepted normal level. The acoustical output, in sound pressure level, required from the earphone to correspond to normal, i.e. 0 dBHL at each frequency, is given in international (and the equivalent British) standards.

The audiogram

This is the graph showing the results obtained in pure tone audiometric testing. Figure 4.1 shows the standard format recommended by the British Society of Audiology. The recommended symbols for use in pure tone audiometry are shown in Figure 4.2. Air-conduction thresholds are represented by circles for the right ear and crosses for the left

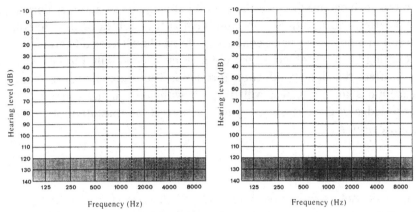

Figure 4.1. Recommended audiogram format.

O Right ear – air conduction

● Right ear – air conduction – not masked (possible shadow threshold)

◖ Right ear – air conduction – masked but no change on masking

X Left ear – air conduction

X̶ Left ear – air conduction – not masked (possible shadow threshold)

X̲ Left ear – air conduction – masked but no change on masking

Δ Bone conduction – not masked

⊏ Right ear – bone conduction

⊐ Left ear – bone conduction

Figure 4.2. Recommended symbols for use in pure tone audiometry.

ear. These measurements are obtained via headphone presentation and thus the signal has to pass through the entire auditory pathway comprising the outer ear, middle ear, inner ear and neural pathways to the auditory cortex before being perceived by the patient. Thus a hearing loss at any stage in this pathway will result in a depressed air-conduction threshold at that frequency. Bone-conduction thresholds are obtained with signals presented via a bone vibrator which is placed on the mastoid process. It is generally assumed that such a signal bypasses the outer and middle ear (the conducting mechanism) and travels directly to the cochlea and then via the neural pathway to the auditory cortex. A hearing loss resulting from a problem at the cochlea or beyond will result in a depressed bone-conduction threshold whereas a hearing loss resulting from a problem in the outer or middle ear will, theoretically, not affect the bone-conduction threshold. There are, however, some exceptions to this, which will be dealt with later in the chapter and knowledge of these is necessary for the correct interpretation of audiometric results.

Calibration

All audiometers should be calibrated and checked at regular intervals to ensure that they comply with the relevant International and British standards. This is obviously important to ensure that results obtained on different audiometers in different settings at different times can be compared accurately.

Threshold measurement

It is important to use a standard recognised technique for the measurement of thresholds so that valid comparison may be made between audiograms obtained at different times by different testers. The threshold measurement procedure may affect the final threshold obtained. A threshold obtained using a descending technique, that is descending from a level that the patient clearly hears until he or she no longer responds, will result in a slightly different threshold from that obtained with an ascending method, that is, ascending from silence and recording the first level at which the patient shows a positive response. There is a signal level at, and above, which a patient will respond on 100% of presentations. Similarly there is a signal level at, and below, which a patient will always fail to respond. In between the two lies the region that contains threshold and the measurement procedure adopted affects the final result obtained.

The method described here is one of the two methods recommended by the British Society of Audiology (British Society of Audiology, 1981, 1985). The first stage involves the familiarisation process where the patient is presented with the tone that is clearly audible and encouraged to make the correct response. Once the patient has demonstrated that he or she understands the task and is able to make the required response, the threshold measurement begins. The signal level is reduced in 10 dB steps until the patient fails to respond and it is then increased in 5 dB steps until the patient again shows a positive response. After such an ascending positive response the level is again reduced in 10 dB steps until a failure to respond and raised in 5 dB steps until a positive response. Threshold is defined as the minimum intensity at which the patient responds on at least 50% of ascending presentations with a minimum of two responses at that level. An example of a threshold tracing is shown in Figure 4.3. This procedure is used to determine air-conduction and bone-conduction thresholds as required.

With older children and adults, verbal instruction and some initial familiarisation are normally all that is required. The response is usually to require the patient to press a button to indicate the onset of the signal and release the button at the offset of the signal. Older children and adults are often tested in sound-proof booths with the tester either inside, or more often outside, the booth. With young children (below 5 years of age) certain modifications to the procedure are normally required in order to maintain the child's cooperation. These measures will be described in the next section.

Signal level (dB)	Patient response at each presentation level (✓ = positive response, X = no response)													
	Start→													End
85														
80														
75														
70	✓													
65														
60		✓												
55														
50			✓											
45														
40				✓										
35						✓*						✓*		
30					X			✓*			X			✓*
25							X			X			X	
20									X					
15														
10														

Threshold = 30 dB

* Ascending positive responses.

Figure 4.3. An example of threshold measurement procedure.

Threshold measurement in children

As with all behavioural methods used for the assessment of hearing in children, the task must be appropriate for the developmental level of the child irrespective of the chronological age. Young children are normally tested in sound-treated rooms or sound-proof booths that are large enough to hold the child, the tester and at least one of the parents as well as the equipment. A suitable arrangement for pure tone audiometry with young children is shown in Figure 4.4. The child is seated on a small chair at a small table with the parent or carer next to the child for reassurance (if necessary the child can also be permitted to sit on the parent's lap for reassurance). The tester is seated or kneels near to the child but with the audiometer out of the child's vision. The tester can then manipulate the dial settings of the audiometer with one hand but at the same time is ideally placed to observe the child's response, to provide praise and encouragement and to maintain the child's attention on the task. The initial phase of testing involves the conditioning procedure whereby the response is demonstrated to the child using clearly suprathreshold signals. This is extremely important as the child cannot be expected to be conditioned to a signal which she

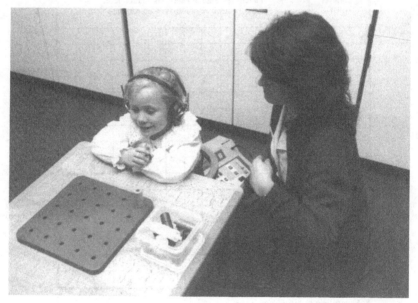

Figure 4.4. Suitable arrangement for pure tone audiometry with a young child.

or he cannot hear. The tester demonstrates the action required upon the presentation of the signal and then guides the child in making the appropriate response when the signal is presented. This initial conditioning is done by demonstration and reward – smiles, words of encouragement – and thus the child is conditioned to perform the task. Complex verbal instructions are avoided so that the child's language level is not a factor in successful conditioning.

The most appropriate response involves the child carrying out a simple motor action, for example placing a peg in a board or a man in a boat, upon presentation of the auditory stimuli. A number of suitable activities of this type should be available. If the child's attention begins to drift then the activity can be exchanged and this is often enough to revive a child's interest in the task. The advantages of this kind of response are:

1. the response itself is interesting and rewarding for the child
2. false positive responses, that is responses in the absence of a signal, can be corrected by the tester, for example by removing the peg from the board
3. simple motor responses involving play materials lend themselves to non-verbal conditioning

It is important that a child is not unduly apprehensive; separation from the parent or caregiver is not advisable and rarely necessary for the purpose of carrying out audiometry with children. The child should be comfortable, freed from other distractions, for example visual distractions within the room should be kept to a minimum, and interruptions should not be permitted. It is also important that background noise does not exceed acceptable levels. Acceptable levels of background noise for diagnostic audiometry are given in the International standards (BS 6655, 1986; ISO 8253-1, 1989). The stringency of the requirement depends upon the lowest threshold level it is desired to measure and the mode of signal presentation, i.e. air-conduction or bone-conduction.

The threshold tracing procedure is essentially the same as that used with adults but it may be necessary to do this at a restricted range of frequencies depending on the child's attention span. This means that the tester may make strategic decisions about which threshold measures to pursue in a given test session. It is sometimes justifiable to test down to a certain level, for instance 15 or 20 dB, rather than spend a lot of time establishing very exact thresholds of –5 or 0 dB. If this is the case this can be indicated appropriately on the audiogram and the threshold recorded as ≤20 dB, for example. The vast majority of normally developing children over the age of 3½ should be able to cooperate, albeit for a limited range of thresholds, with pure tone audiometric testing if the tester is sufficiently skilled. Between the ages of 2½ and 3½ an increasing number of children should also be able to cooperate with this procedure.

Interpretation of audiograms

Pure tone audiometry can provide a great deal of information about a patient's hearing because:

1. It is usually possible to assess accurately the hearing in each ear independently although in certain cases it may be necessary to use a technique called masking to achieve this.
2. Comparison of air- and bone-conduction thresholds for each ear provides a measure of the air–bone gap and thus of any conductive component to the hearing loss.

If pure tone audiometry merely involved obtaining threshold measurements with a headphone and a bone vibrator for each ear, then it would be a relatively straightforward task. However, one of the major problems in obtaining valid pure tone audiograms arises from the ability of sound to cross the head and reach the contralateral (i.e. opposite) ear. If a sound presented to one ear, the test ear, is sufficiently intense, it may cross the skull and be perceived in the cochlea of the non-test ear. If the patient responds positively to this signal a false threshold will be recorded for the test ear. The crucial factors in determining whether this 'cross-hearing' is likely to be occurring are:

1. the intensity of the signal presented to the test ear
2. the amount of sound energy lost in crossing the skull (the transcranial attenuation)
3. the hearing sensitivity of the contralateral, i.e. non-test cochlea

For air-conduction stimuli presented via conventional headphones, the minimum value of transcranial attenuation is 40 dB. Thus, if any air-conduction threshold is found to be greater than the contralateral bone-conduction threshold by 40 dB or more, there is the possibility that cross-hearing is occurring, i.e. the sound being presented to the test ear has crossed the skull and is being perceived in the non-test cochlea.

For bone-conduction stimuli the minimum value of transcranial attenuation is 0 dB. Thus any bone-conduction threshold obtained without masking cannot with certainty be ascribed to a particular cochlea. If the bone vibrator is placed on the right mastoid this does not necessarily mean that the threshold obtained reflects the sensitivity of the right cochlea. All that can be said is that it reflects the sensitivity of the better cochlea.

Masking

In order to overcome the problems of cross-hearing a technique known as masking is used. This involves presenting a noise (usually a narrow band noise centred on the test frequency) to the non-test ear in order to 'occupy' it whilst at the same time remeasuring the threshold in the test ear. It will be obvious that there is then a possibility that the masking noise may in turn cross over and affect the threshold in the test ear. This is known as cross-masking. It is necessary to ensure that the correct level of masking is used; too little masking will not prevent the non-test ear from responding to the threshold measurement; too much masking will cross over and artificially raise the threshold in the test ear. In order to achieve this correct level of masking it is necessary to increase the masking level in discrete steps and at each level to remeasure the test ear threshold. Standard procedures for masked threshold determination have been agreed by the British Society of Audiology (British Society of Audiology, 1986). It is not appropriate here to go into further details of this procedure but interested readers are referred to Wood (1993).

It will be obvious that this can be a time consuming procedure that requires a thorough knowledge on the part of the tester as well as experience in carrying this out with young children. The age at which reliable masked threshold measurement can be undertaken is quite variable but many children of 4 years of age and above can cooperate with this task for a limited period. In these cases the tester must make strategic decisions based upon the information available as to which masked thresholds should be obtained as a matter of priority.

Examples

The following examples illustrate some of the problems involved in the correct interpretation of audiometric results. In each case the not-masked air-conduction thresholds are shown followed, where appropriate, by the not-masked bone-conduction thresholds. The necessity for further masked threshold determination is then discussed along with some possible results.

Example 1: In this example, the audiogram in Figure 4.5 shows that the air-conduction thresholds are within normal limits in both ears. There is no indication to carry out any bone-conduction threshold measurement as this will not add any further useful information. The bone-conduction thresholds are always, at least theoretically, as good as or better than the air-conduction thresholds and therefore, in this case, they too will be within the normal range.

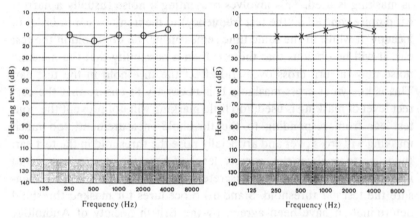

Figure 4.5. Audiogram showing normal hearing in both ears.

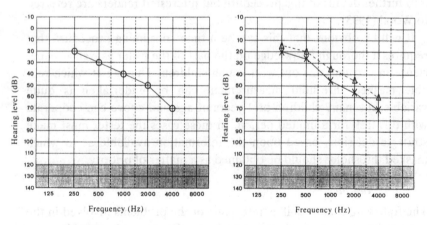

Figure 4.6. Audiogram showing a bilateral high frequency sensorineural loss.

Example 2: In this example, illustrated in Figure 4.6, the air-conduction thresholds show a symmetrical bilateral sloping hearing loss that is more marked at higher frequencies. The bone-conduction thresholds (obtained without masking) show a similar pattern. Although it is not possible to say for certain which cochlea is responding it is possible to say that, whichever it is, there is no possibility of a significant air–bone gap in either ear. Therefore, no further useful information would be obtained by carrying out masked bone-conduction threshold measurement for each ear separately. Generally an air–bone gap of 15 dB or more is regarded as significant.

Example 3: In this example the not-masked air-conduction audiogram is given in Figure 4.7 and shows a symmetrical bilateral loss but this time with a flat configuration. Clearly there is a significant hearing loss and further assessment is necessary to ascertain whether there may be a conductive factor present. The first step would again be to obtain the not-masked bone-conduction thresholds.

Suppose this produced the result shown in Figure 4.8. Again, it is possible to state that although we do not know for certain which cochlea is responding there is no possibility of a significant air–bone gap in either ear and therefore the results confirm a mild bilateral sensorineural hearing loss.

However, if the bone-conduction thresholds were found to be as shown in Figure 4.9 then this would be a very different (and in children a much more common) situation. In this case the bone-conduction thresholds tell us that the hearing in the better cochlea is normal irre-

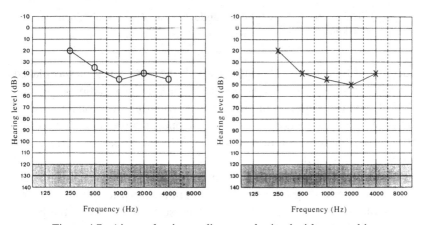

Figure 4.7. Air-conduction audiogram obtained without masking.

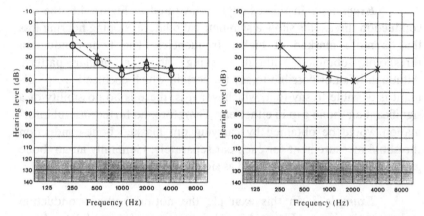

Figure 4.8. Audiogram showing a bilateral flat sensorineural hearing loss.

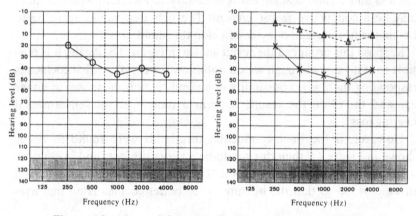

Figure 4.9. Air- and bone-conduction audiogram obtained without masking.

spective of the side of the head on which the bone vibrator was placed for the measurement. In order to obtain further information about the size of any air–bone gap in either ear it would be necessary to obtain masked bone-conduction thresholds for one or both ears. If the child truly had a bilateral conductive hearing loss this would give the results shown in Figure 4.10.

However, it is possible that a number of other configurations of hearing loss could have produced the audiogram shown in Figure 4.9. The bone-conduction thresholds in one ear must be at or around the levels obtained without masking but the loss in the other ear could be entirely

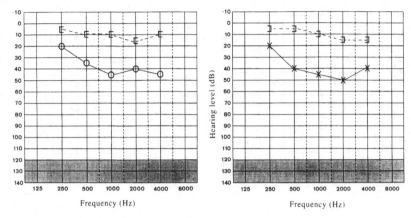

Figure 4.10. Audiogram showing a bilateral conductive hearing loss.

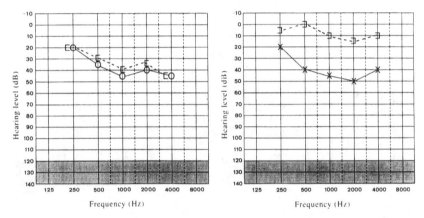

Figure 4.11. Audiogram showing a right-sided sensorineural loss and a left-sided conductive loss.

sensorineural as shown in Figure 4.11. Equally, it could be that there is a mixed loss in the right ear with a conductive loss in the left as shown in Figure 4.12.

In all the previous examples, although bone-conduction masking has often been necessary to measure the air–bone gap accurately, no air-conduction masking has been required. Examination of all the previous audiograms shows that there has been no marked asymmetry in the not-masked air-conduction thresholds and in the cases where masked bone-conduction threshold measurement has been carried out there is no case where the gap between an air-conduction threshold and the true

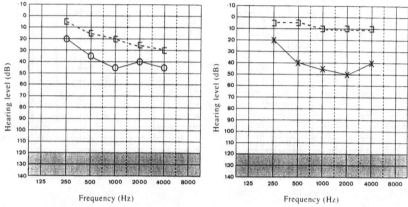

Figure 4.12. Audiogram showing a right-sided mixed loss and a left-sided conductive loss.

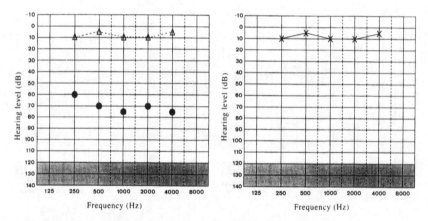

Figure 4.13. Audiogram obtained without masking.

(i.e. masked) contralateral bone-conduction threshold has exceeded 40 dB. In the next example there is clearly a possibility of cross-hearing for both air- and bone-conduction thresholds and masking is required for both.

Example 4: The audiogram shown in Figure 4.13 shows normal air-conduction thresholds for the left ear with thresholds depressed at around the 60 dB level in the right ear. The not-masked bone-conduction thresholds are bound to be within the normal range since we already know from the air-conduction audiogram that the left ear has normal hearing. In order to obtain the true bone-conduction thresholds for the right ear it will be necessary to use masking. Having done this, there is still clearly the possibility that the air-conduction thresholds for the right ear are 'shadow' thresholds resulting from the sound crossing over the head and being perceived in the left, or non-test, cochlea. In order to eliminate this possibility it will be necessary to redetermine the right-ear air-conduction thresholds with masking in the left ear.

Figures 4.14 and 4.15 show two possible audiometric configurations that would initially produce the not-masked audiogram shown in Figure 4.13. In the case illustrated in Figure 4.14 it can be seen that once masking is introduced, the right cochlea fails to respond at the maximum output of the bone conductor and this is indicated by downward arrows on

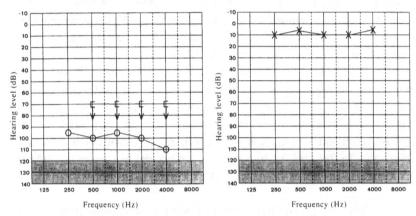

Figure 4.14. Audiogram showing normal hearing in the left ear and a severe loss in the right ear.

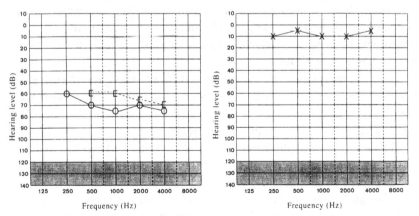

Figure 4.15. Audiogram showing normal hearing in the left ear and a moderate sensorineural loss in the right ear.

the audiogram at the maximum output levels. Furthermore, when masking is used in order to redetermine the right-ear air-conduction thresholds the true thresholds are shifted considerably, indicating that the original thresholds recorded were 'shadow' thresholds resulting from cross-hearing. In this case the true picture is of a profound sensorineural loss in the right ear with normal hearing in the left ear. Clearly the bone-conduction thresholds for the right ear cannot be determined and therefore information about the existence of any conductive component to the hearing loss in the right ear will need to be obtained by other means, e.g. impedance measurements (Chapter 6) and/or clinical examination (Chapter 2).

Figure 4.15 illustrates another audiometric configuration that could produce the audiogram shown in Figure 4.13. In this case the masked bone-conduction thresholds for the right ear are shown. There is still a requirement for masking of the right-ear air-conduction thresholds but when this is carried out there is no appreciable shift of the thresholds obtained. Therefore, in this case the original not-masked right-ear air-conduction thresholds were not a result of cross-hearing and were valid. However, because of the individual variability in the transcranial attenuation, it was not possible to predict this result and masking was necessary in order to ensure that the results were valid. In this case the true picture is of normal hearing in the left ear with a moderate sensorineural loss in the right ear.

Example 5: Another problem that may sometimes arise in pure tone audiometry, particularly with children with severe or profound hearing loss, is the possibility that the child is responding to the vibratory rather than the auditory content of a signal. This may occur at frequencies up to and including 1 kHz and can occur at relatively low output levels for bone-conduction stimuli but only at high output levels for air-conduction stimuli.

Given the audiogram shown in Figure 4.16, the naive tester may well interpret this as showing a severe bilateral sensorineural loss with the possibility of a significant air–bone gap at low frequencies, thus indicating a conductive component to the hearing loss. In fact the bone-conduction thresholds shown at 250 Hz, 500 Hz and 1 kHz could well be the result of vibratory rather than auditory sensation and, therefore, do not give any useful information about the hearing.

In the audiogram in Figure 4.17 all the thresholds shown, both air- and bone-conduction, could be the result of vibrotactile rather than auditory perception. Again, there is a considerable amount of individ-

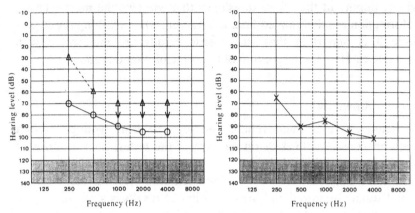

Figure 4.16. Audiogram showing vibrotactile bone-conduction thresholds.

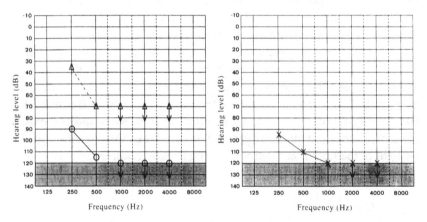

Figure 4.17. Audiogram showing vibrotactile air- and bone-conduction thresholds.

ual variability in the levels at which vibrotactile perception occurs and it is not possible to state with certainty that this is occurring but rather to bear in mind the possibility that this may be the case.

Use of masking with children

From the examples discussed above it will be clear that obtaining full masked audiograms can be a time consuming procedure requiring considerable cooperation from the patient. When testing young children it is often not possible to obtain comprehensive results and, therefore, it is vitally important that those thresholds that will give the most relevant information are determined first. In addition, when masking is not possible it is important that audiometric results are interpreted with extreme caution, taking account of the principles set out above.

Summary

Obtaining accurate and reliable audiograms from young children requires considerable skills on the part of the tester, both in terms of child-handling skills and also in interpreting the results obtained.

In cases of symmetrical bilateral sensorineural hearing loss, masking is not usually required and interpretation of results is straightforward. In cases of asymmetric and/or conductive hearing loss careful interpretation is needed and masked threshold measurement may be required. This may not be possible in young children and it is, therefore, important to have a clear understanding of the limitations of the information obtained when interpreting audiometric results.

In general, when an audiogram is obtained without masking, the better-ear air-conduction thresholds will be accurate and the bone-conduction thresholds will reflect the status of the better cochlea (although this may not be the same ear as the better-ear air-conduction thresholds). The validity of the worse-ear air-conduction thresholds and the existence of a significant air–bone gap will need to be evaluated carefully in the light of the potential for cross-hearing to have occurred.

References

British Society of Audiology (1981). Recommended procedures for pure tone audiometry using a manually operated instrument. *British Journal of Audiology*, **15**, 213–16.

British Society of Audiology (1985). Recommended procedures for pure tone bone conduction audiometry without masking using a manually operated instrument. *British Journal of Audiology*, **19**, 281–2.

British Society of Audiology (1986). Recommendations for masking in pure tone threshold audiometry. *British Journal of Audiology*, **20**, 307–14.

BS 6655 (1986). *Pure Tone Air Conduction Threshold Audiometry for Hearing Conservation Purposes*. London: British Standards Institution.

ISO (1989). *Acoustics – Audiometric Test Methods – Part 1: Basic Pure Tone Air and Bone Conduction Threshold Audiometry, ISO 8253-1*. Geneva: International Organisation for Standardisation.

Wood, S. (1993). Pure tone audiometry. In *Paediatric Audiology, 0–5 years*, 2nd edn (ed. B. McCormick), pp. 155–86. London: Whurr Publishers Limited.

5

Objective hearing tests

YVONNE COPE

Introduction

Audiological test methods, like various other clinical investigations, can be categorised into behavioural, subjective and objective techniques. The behavioural and subjective classes are often grouped as one.

Behavioural

These methods involve monitoring the patients' reactions to auditory stimuli. The response may be involuntary, e.g. when using the distraction technique an infant will instinctively turn to locate a sound of interest. It may also be voluntary; the more mature child undergoing distraction testing may elect to inhibit his or her response.

Subjective

These methods require the patient to volunteer a response, such as in pure tone or speech audiometry.

Objective

These methods require no voluntary indication from the patient that an auditory stimulus has been perceived. It is possible, however, for the patient to influence the results by interfering with the procedure. In a sense, the subjectivity is transferred to the clinician, who in many cases interprets the results, although machine scoring methods are being used increasingly. Objective tests are not a measure of hearing as such; they assess the integrity at various levels of the auditory pathway but not its entirety.

This chapter is devoted to a description of two objective measurements widely used in paediatric audiology, the auditory brainstem response (ABR) and the delayed evoked otoacoustic emission. The basic principles, measurement techniques, result interpretation and applications will be discussed.

The auditory brainstem response

In response to auditory stimulation it is possible to evoke electrical impulses at various levels along the length of the auditory pathway and these are known as auditory evoked potentials (AEPs). These potentials are recorded as the differential signal between a pair of surface scalp electrodes. The ABR is just one of these potentials and the term generally given to the measurement technique is electric response audiometry (ERA).

The measurement of AEPs advanced in the 1950s following the development of signal averaging techniques and the electronic digital averaging computer, pioneered by Dawson (1951) and Clark (1958) respectively. It became possible to extract and measure the tiny AEPs, with amplitudes in the microvolt range, differentiating them from the larger contaminating signals produced by general muscular and electroencephalographic (EEG) activity. It was as recently as the 1970s that the first definitive description of the ABR appeared in the paper by Jewitt and Williston (1971), although it was Sohmer and Feinmesser (1967) who first recorded the response. Davis (1976) and Gibson (1978) have reviewed the historical development of AEPs.

Classification of AEPs

As mentioned earlier, it is possible to measure AEPs along the entire length of the auditory pathway, originating from the hair cells of the cochlea, the auditory nerve, the brainstem and the auditory cortex up to and including the cerebral cortex. Classification is a complex subject and far beyond the scope of this chapter; Davis (1976) has discussed this topic in detail. It is important, however, to appreciate the classification usually assigned to a particular AEP. The two most commonly used descriptions refer to:

1. the physiological site of generation, either neurogenic or myogenic

2. the response latency, either early, middle or late, depending on the time the response occurs after the stimulus

The ABR is of neural origin, in the auditory nerve and brainstem pathways, and early latency, occurring within the first 10 ms after the stimulus.

Choice of AEP

There are many options within ERA; each AEP has its own strengths and weaknesses dependent on the required application, e.g. screening, threshold estimation or the assessment of cochlear and retrocochlear pathology. Additionally, practicalities such as the test facilities, staffing and tester skills, behavioural state of the patient, the effect of sedation or anaesthesia on the AEP need to be considered. These aspects have been discussed in greater detail by a number of authors, e.g. Gibson (1978) and Mason (1993).

The primary practice for ERA in children is aimed at the estimation of the hearing threshold when conventional audiological techniques are unreliable or cannot be carried out. It is the ABR that has achieved prominence for this purpose. The assessment of the integrity of the central auditory pathway is a different, albeit equally important, matter reserved for differential diagnostic cases.

Origin and configuration of the ABR waveform

Typically the ABR waveform comprises a series of up to eight identifiable components, waves I to VII and a negative trough, the SN10, occurring at about 10 ms post-stimulus time (see Figure 5.1). In the newborn population the waveform is somewhat different; it usually comprises just three identifiable wave peaks, I, III and V, the latency is greater and the amplitude differs from that of the more mature response. Several factors are thought to be responsible for the latency change, e.g. cochlear immaturity and the extent to which the nerve fibres are myelinated.

The anatomical origin of many of the AEPs is still uncertain. There exists, however, reasonable evidence to suggest that components I to VII of the ABR originate from peripheral nerves and more central auditory pathways (see Table 5.1). The SN10 component is thought to originate from the midbrain (Davis and Hirsh, 1979).

Table 5.1 *Wave I to VII complex*

	Origin
Waves I and II	Auditory nerve
Wave III	Cochlear nucleus
Wave IV	Superior olivary complex
Wave V	Lateral lemniscus
Wave VI and VII	Inferior colliculus

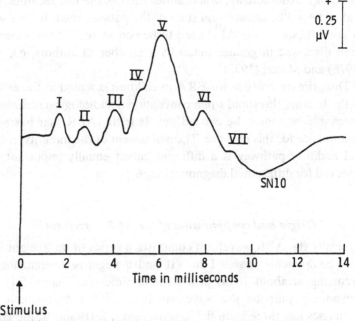

Figure 5.1. Components of the ABR. Based on Figure 7.18 of the article by Mason (1993).

Recording the ABR

Recording the ABR is a non-invasive, painless procedure. It is unaffected by sleep or sedation and if the recording conditions are good the test duration can be reasonably short, typically 20–30 minutes.

The evoked potential is measured as the differential signal across a pair of electrodes. An active electrode is positioned over an area of high response activity, the vertex of the scalp, and a reference electrode is positioned over an area of low response, often the earlobe or mastoid bone of the test ear. A third electrode, acting as the earth, is positioned on the forehead. The electrodes are non-invasive, surface type, of a similar configuration to the standard EEG electrode. Prior to application, the skin surface is cleaned with surgical spirit and to obtain good contact between the skin and electrode a conductive jelly is applied. The patient is settled, ideally sitting quietly or in a state of sleep before recording commences (Figure 5.2). Technological advancements have resulted in the size of the equipment being scaled down over recent years.

The following is a brief summary of the instrumentation required and recording methodology usually adopted; Mason (1993) has described this in detail. A controlled acoustical stimulus, which is often a sharp click-type sound, is delivered to the ear under test through an earphone or a transducer, modified for small infants. This produces a synchro-

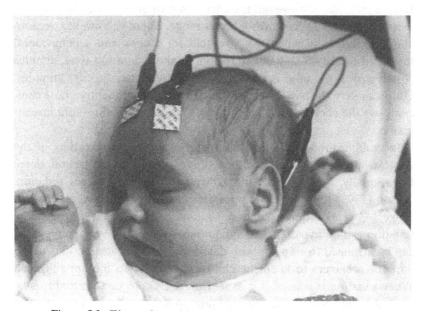

Figure 5.2. Electrode positions for recording the ABR in a neonate. A good contact at the vertex is occasionally difficult to achieve with the delicate fontanelle in very young babies and the active electrode is routinely positioned at a high forehead site.

nised discharge in the auditory system, which is detected by the recording electrodes. The signal comprises not only the AEP but also electrical background noise, EEG, heart and myogenic activity. A differential amplifier enhances the weak AEP and suppresses, to a certain extent, the unwanted noise. Filtering is used to eliminate any frequency components within the signal that do not correlate with the response of interest, and signal averaging further enhances the AEP. The amplified signal from the electrodes is sampled over a given time period immediately after the stimulus, a sweep. Typically 2000 to 4000 individual sweeps are sampled, summed and averaged depending on the recording conditions. The AEP waveform does not vary significantly during the averaging process of the individual sweeps, unlike the random background noise. As the number of sampled sweeps increases, the AEP superimposes and becomes better defined. The background noise activity will cancel out.

The stimuli are of a different characteristic to those used in conventional pure tone audiometry. A stimulus of fast onset/offset is required so as to produce good synchronisation of the firing of nerve fibres that results in a well-defined ABR waveform. A click is typically used. Unlike pure tones, however, the click is not frequency specific and possesses acoustical energy over a broad range. There is, however, reasonable correlation between the threshold for a click and a behavioural threshold in the 2000–4000 Hz region. A short duration tone stimulus (tone pip) is an alternative and more frequency-specific stimulus. Unfortunately the ABR is less well defined. Consequently, most clinicians use the click as their first choice of stimulus for threshold investigation.

In most instances it is possible to make a reliable recording of the ABR whilst the patient is either sitting quietly or in natural sleep. Occasionally, however, it is necessary to administer a light sedation. Mason (1993) reported that approximately 30% of children in the age range 1–3 years require sedation. In most cases, with careful planning, sedation can be avoided. The appointment time for a very young child can be arranged to coincide with daytime sleep, with instructions to the parents/caregivers to keep the child awake prior to the appointment. When sedation is needed it is usual for the child to be admitted to hospital the day before the investigation to undergo a general medical assessment.

Interpretation of results

The aim in threshold investigation is to measure the lowest level of stimulus required to evoke the ABR. It is usually the wave V and SN10 components that remain identifiable down to threshold level (Figure 5.3).

Typically, the dB step size is larger than in conventional audiometry. Initially steps of 20 dB are used, then when the response waveform appears to be approaching threshold, the step size is reduced to 10 dB.

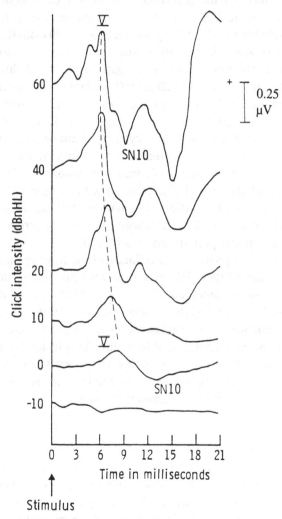

Figure 5.3. ABR waveforms recorded down to hearing threshold in a normally hearing child.

The dB scale differs from that used in subjective audiometry. The stimulus is calibrated in dB above the hearing threshold of normally hearing subjects and is given the notation dBnHL. The accuracy of threshold prediction is dependent on a number of factors, e.g. the recording conditions and skill of the tester. Response identification is a highly skilled procedure and in most cases is performed subjectively. Techniques of machine scoring to assist with the task are now in existence (Mason, 1993). Mason (1985) reported the ABR threshold to be usually within 10 dB of the behavioural threshold for mature subjects or a child sitting quietly for the test. Even for very young babies the click-evoked ABR can be reliably recorded down to levels below 20 dBnHL. In premature babies the ABR is immature and may result in raised thresholds (Mason, 1993). For routine investigations a normal threshold for the click is usually reported as 20 dBnHL or better. This does not however imply that thresholds for all frequencies of sound are within normal limits. Due to the lack of frequency specificity of the click ABR, the hearing sensitivity in certain frequency regions can be overestimated and it is possible to overlook an area of hearing impairment. An audiogram with a sloping or notched configuration may not be estimated correctly. Results must therefore be interpreted with caution and always alongside behavioural observations. Behavioural methods are much less time consuming and provide much more information across the frequency range if a response pattern can be achieved.

In addition to providing an estimate of the hearing threshold, certain characteristics of the ABR waveform may provide an indication as to whether a hearing loss is cochlear, retrocochlear or conductive in origin. Occasionally, ABR threshold measurement with stimuli delivered via a bone-conduction transducer is used to determine whether a hearing loss is conductive or sensorineural in nature. This is, however, problematic due to the poor frequency-response characteristics of the transducer, the consistency of coupling the bone-conduction transducer to the head and the presence of a large stimulus artefact.

The delayed evoked otoacoustic emission

Otoacoustic emissions (OAEs) are the release of low-intensity sound energy, generated by the cochlea and measurable within the external auditory meatus. They are a relatively recent discovery and were first recognised by Kemp (1978). Following the presentation of an acoustic stimulus to the ear and with the aid of a sensitive miniature microphone sealed in the external auditory meatus, he recorded a brief, low-intensity acoustic response generated by the cochlea, the delayed evoked OAE.

Classification of OAEs

The delayed evoked OAE is just one of four distinct but interrelated categories, the others being the spontaneous, the simultaneous and the distortion product OAE. The distinguishing factor is the method used to evoke and record them. The spontaneous emission requires no stimulation at all and is present in approximately 30–60% of all normal human ears. The remaining three categories all require a stimulus to evoke them and are present in the vast majority of all normal ears. The simultaneous OAE arises as the synchronous response to a continuous tonal stimulus and usually manifests as an interaction between the stimulus and the OAE. Distortion product OAEs are the product of the simultaneous presentation of two continuous tones at closely spaced frequencies. The OAE can be measured at intermodulation frequencies of the stimuli. The delayed evoked OAE arises immediately after the presentation of a brief acoustic stimulus, such as a click or tone burst. For a description of each category of OAE the reader may wish to refer to Probst, Lonsbury-Martin and Martin (1991) and Cope and Lutman (1993).

Choice of OAE

For a number of reasons it is the delayed evoked OAE that clinically has proven to be the most useful in paediatric audiology, particularly in the screening context. There is general agreement that it shows a uniform behaviour in the vast majority of the population with normal hearing and is produced only in the presence of a healthy or at least partially healthy cochlea and middle ear.

Origin and configuration of the delayed evoked OAE

There is now agreement that OAEs originate from the cochlea and that evoked OAEs, and in most cases spontaneous OAEs, are consistent with the presence of normal mechanically active functioning of the outer hair cells within the cochlea.

The features of the delayed evoked OAE have been extensively investigated; Probst *et al.* (1991) have comprehensively reviewed much of the experimental work. Basically, the response waveform is divisible into two distinct parts (Figure 5.4). Each part behaves differently with increasing levels of stimulation. The first part increases linearly with increasing levels of stimulus, whereas the second part exhibits a non-linear growth with increasing stimulus level. It is this contrasting behaviour that partly distinguishes the initial artefactual component from the later OAE. The OAE is much smaller in amplitude than the artefact and each ear has its own characteristic pattern of response but generally has the appearance of a burst of oscillation (Figure 5.5). They are very stable over periods of time and have a frequency content within the 500–4000 Hz range. They are altered or abolished by middle-ear impairment and are absent when the hearing impairment is in excess of 20–25 dBHL.

Recording the delayed evoked OAE

Recording the delayed evoked OAE is a non-invasive procedure with no discomfort to the patient. If recording conditions are good, ideally the child is quiet or asleep, a recording from one ear can be made in approximately 1 minute. If the child becomes active, the results are less reliable. It is usual, therefore, for the test to be stopped during active periods and restarted when the child has settled, thus increasing the test time. Recent work undertaken by Thornton (1993) using increased

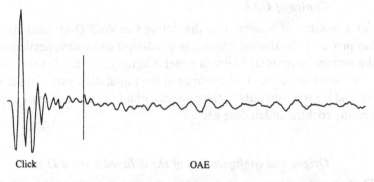

Click   OAE

Figure 5.4. Recording of a typical delayed evoked OAE following click stimulation. The early part of the trace is the acoustical response of the ear and measurement system to the click stimulus and is mainly due to the ringing of the transducers. The remainder of the trace (amplified by a factor of 32 relative to the earlier part) is the click-evoked OAE. From Cope and Lutman (1993).

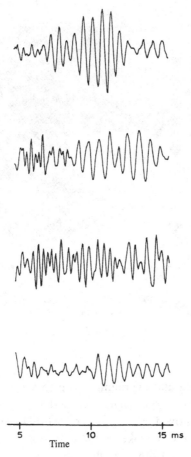

Figure 5.5. Delayed evoked OAEs, following click stimulation, recorded from adults with normal hearing. Note the inter-subject variation in waveform morphology. Based on Figure 8.9 of the article by Cope and Lutman (1993).

rates of stimulus presentation has the potential to significantly reduce the test time, to seconds rather than minutes.

The equipment required to record an OAE comprises an acoustic probe, inserted into the patient's external auditory meatus and sealed with the aid of a replaceable soft plastic cuff (Figure 5.6). The probe houses a miniature loudspeaker and microphone for stimulus delivery and response capture respectively. Additionally, there is a narrow-bore vent to allow for pressure equalisation.

OAEs are of a very low amplitude, typically less than 20 dBSPL, and easily masked by extraneous noise. Therefore to enhance the signal-to-

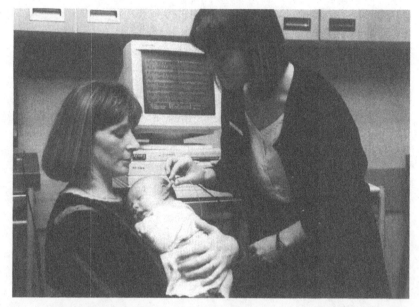

Figure 5.6. Probe placement for recording the delayed evoked OAE in a young baby.

noise ratio filtering and averaging of up to several hundred responses are employed. Interfering signals caused by swallowing and general movement are removed by a method of overload rejection.

The stimulus used to evoke an OAE is of a short duration, such as a click or tone burst. Both stimuli excite the same OAE generating process. Tone burst stimuli have the potential to provide more frequency-specific information but the click, albeit less frequency specific, remains the stimulus most widely used and existing knowledge is based mostly on data using clicks.

Response identification is a skilled procedure and is assisted by examining several features of the OAE waveform. Automatic scoring methods based, for example, on calculation of the cross-correlation of replicate waveforms, have also been developed (Lutman, 1993).

Result interpretation

The presence of an OAE is consistent with normal or near to normal cochlear function which, provided there is no retrocochlear dysfunction, is compatible with normal or near to normal hearing at least at some frequencies. Click-evoked OAEs are usually absent if the hearing level exceeds 20–25 dB. It is therefore not possible to determine the degree or configuration of hearing impairment from click-evoked OAE measures alone and behavioural techniques or other objective tests such as ABR threshold investigation must be used. OAEs are also absent in the presence of middle-ear abnormality such as otitis media with effusion. Thus it is important to rule out the presence of a middle-ear disorder if an individual does not possess an OAE. A small minority of individuals with normal hearing do not exhibit OAEs. This may be a consequence of the properties of the individual's middle or outer ears, or poor recording conditions; the OAE is of a very small amplitude and is easily masked by larger ambient noise components. As with ABR measurements it is important to interpret OAE test results in conjunction with behavioural observations.

Clinical applications of the ABR and delayed evoked OAE

Both the ABR and delayed evoked OAE are valuable in the audiological assessment of the very young or otherwise difficult to assess child. The two tests are quite different and have advantages and limitations depending on the required application, either screening or diagnostic. The OAE test is specific to cochlear function, is very fast and in most cases its presence is consistent with hearing levels better than 25 dBHL, for some frequencies at least. When the hearing level is in excess of about 25 dBHL or there is a conductive element, the OAE will be absent and it is not possible to obtain any further information about the degree of hearing loss from OAE measurements alone. Measurement of the ABR is a longer procedure. Quantitatively, however, the ABR provides more information regarding the hearing level. It covers the entire audible range for intensity, thus documenting hearing loss from mild to profound.

Screening

It is a well recognised aim to detect significant hearing impairment at the earliest stage possible. Work on auditory deprivation has shown that the earlier a hearing loss is quantified and management initiated the greater is the communicative ability (Ramkalawan and Davis, 1992). Depending on a number of factors it may be neither practical nor possible to screen every live birth for hearing impairment and therefore targeted groups at greater risk for hearing impairment may be screened. In the UK, figures suggest that for the general population the incidence of severe to profound sensorineural hearing loss is of the order of 1 or 2 per 1000. Babies requiring special care in the neonatal period can be up to ten times more likely to have a significant bilateral impairment (Davis and Wood, 1992). Both the ABR and click evoked OAE methods have been subject to many trials and both methods are feasible as a neonatal screen.

Diagnostic

Within paediatric audiology there is always a group of children who defy the skills and expertise of even the most experienced clinician. These children may have physical, neurological or intellectual deficits and although it may be possible to gain some information from behavioural techniques, objective techniques may help to complete the picture.

Other children requiring objective assessment include those presenting with suspected non-organic hearing loss, that is those who feign or exaggerate hearing loss on subjective audiometry. This may be deliberate or unconscious and associated with physical or emotional disorders. ABR threshold investigation may provide a quantitative estimate of the true hearing level with respect to the exaggerated subjective hearing threshold.

Another important group is infants whose parents suspect hearing loss from an early age and when they are not developmentally ready for distraction assessment or where behavioural observation is not conclusive or raises cause for concern. Objective tests may be used to investigate the auditory function.

Cochlear implant patients

ABR and delayed evoked OAE measurements are used as a part of the audiological test battery for the assessment of children undergoing evaluation for cochlear implantation. ABR measurements are used routinely to confirm objectively the degree of hearing loss and delayed evoked OAE measurements have a role in assessing cochlear function. ABR measurements are also used to assess the cochlear implant function following surgery (Mason, 1993). The integrity of the implanted electrodes is assessed by electrically stimulating the electrodes and measuring the brainstem response; because of the nature of the stimulus the measurement is termed the electrical ABR (EABR). In addition to confirming the integrity of the implant, the EABR threshold can be used to predict the subjective electrical threshold, i.e. the level of electrical stimulation the patient requires to perceive the stimulus. This is beneficial for device switch-on and tuning in young children (Sheppard, 1993).

Summary

Objective tests are a valuable assessment tool in paediatric audiology and it is without doubt that they have allowed for previously difficult-to-assess groups to undergo prompt audiological evaluation. The ABR and measurement of the delayed evoked OAE have proven particularly useful for clinicians working in paediatric audiology. In most cases, the ability to detect a delayed evoked OAE or measure an ABR threshold at 20 dBnHL is consistent with normal or near to normal auditory function at certain frequencies. Hearing is, however, a perceptual process and the reader will appreciate that objective tests are not a measure of hearing as such. They assess the integrity at various levels of the auditory pathway but not its entirety. The results of objective tests should therefore always be interpreted with some degree of caution and in conjunction with observations of the patient's behavioural auditory performance. When used in this context objective and behavioural techniques act as complementary tools in the overall assessment.

References

Clark, W. A. Jr (1958). *Average response computer (ARC-1)*. Quarterly Progress Report No. 49, Research Laboratory of Electronics, Massachusetts Institute of Technology, Cambridge, Massachusetts. Cambridge, MA: MIT Press.

Cope, Y. and Lutman, M. E. (1993). Otoacoustic emissions. In *Paediatric Audiology 0–5 Years*, 2nd edn (ed. B. McCormick), pp. 250–90. London: Whurr Publishers Limited.

Davis, A. C. and Wood, S. (1992). The epidemiology of childhood hearing impairment: factors relevant to planning of services. *British Journal of Audiology*, **26**, 77–90.

Davis, H. (1976). Principles of electric response audiometry. *Annals of Otology, Rhinology and Laryngology*, **85**, (Supplement 28), 1–96.

Davis, H. and Hirsh, S. K. (1979). A slow brainstem response for low-frequency audiometry. *Audiology*, **18**, 445–61.

Dawson, G. D. (1951). A summation technique for detecting small signals in a large irregular background. *Journal of Physiology*, **115**, 2–3.

Gibson, W. P. R. (1978). *Essentials of Clinical Electric Response Audiometry*. London: Churchill Livingstone.

Jewitt, D. L. and Williston, J. S. (1971). Auditory-evoked far fields averaged from the scalp of humans. *Brain*, **94**, 681–96.

Kemp, D. T. (1978). Stimulated acoustic emissions from within the human auditory system. *Journal of the Acoustical Society of America*, **64**, 1386–91.

Lutman, M. E. (1993). Reliable identification of click-evoked otoacoustic emissions using signal-processing techniques. *British Journal of Audiology*, **27**, 103–8.

Mason, S. M. (1985). Objective waveform detection in electric response audiometry. PhD thesis, University of Nottingham.

Mason, S. M. (1993). Electric response audiometry. In *Paediatric Audiology 0–5 Years*, 2nd edn (ed. B. McCormick), pp. 187–249. London: Whurr Publishers Limited.

Probst, R., Lonsbury-Martin, B. L. and Martin, G. K. (1991). A review of otoacoustic emissions. *Journal of the Acoustical Society of America*, **89**, 2027–67.

Ramkalawan, T. W. and Davis, A. C. (1992). The effects of hearing loss and age of intervention on some language metrics in young hearing-impaired children. *British Journal of Audiology*, **26**, 97–108.

Sheppard, S. (1993) Cochlear implants. In *Paediatric Audiology 0–5 Years*, 2nd edn (ed. B. McCormick), pp. 402–36. London: Whurr Publishers Limited.

Sohmer, H. and Feinmesser, M. (1967). Cochlear action potentials recorded from the external ear in man. *Annals of Otology, Rhinology and Laryngology*, **76**, 427–35.

Thornton, A. R. D. (1993). Click-evoked otoacoustic emissions: new techniques and applications. *British Journal of Audiology*, **27**, 109–16.

6
Middle-ear measurements
CATHERINE COTTINGHAM

The need for middle-ear measurements

Tympanometry and middle-ear measurements provide important information about the pathological state of the middle ear. The amount of information to be gained from otoscopy alone is dependent on the skill and experience of the clinician and is variable. Audiological tests are also limited in the information they provide about the middle ear. Behavioural audiological tests give information about air-conduction thresholds only. Full audiometry provides only inferential information about the state of the middle ear when air- and bone-conduction thresholds are compared. Even in cases where an air–bone gap is apparent, audiometry alone gives no information about the reasons for this. Audiometric measurements are subjective and rely on the cooperation of the patient. Tympanometry and middle-ear measurements provide a quick method for obtaining objective information about the middle ear and should be included routinely within the audiological test battery.

Underlying principles of middle-ear impedance

Sound, in the form of longitudinal sound waves, may be propagated through solids, liquids and gases. When the sound waves meet a change in medium, the efficiency of propagation is affected. This change in medium causes some sound waves to be transmitted further, or absorbed and some to be reflected back depending on the different characteristic impedances of the different media. Air has a low, and water has a high characteristic impedance. The middle ear acts as an acoustical transformer to overcome the problem of energy loss due to this impedance mismatch between the air in the ear canal and the fluid in the cochlea.

The middle-ear structures have properties of mass, elasticity and friction. Changes in these properties normally have an adverse effect on the system and therefore measurements of such changes are of clinical interest.

Middle-ear measurement systems

Middle-ear measurement systems may be known as: middle-ear analysers, impedance meters, immitance meters, or otoadmittance meters. Although all these systems perform similar functions, they may differ in other aspects, such as their degree of automation. They may also differ in complexity according to whether it is a screening or diagnostic system. As with most equipment, it is important to choose a particular model according to the needs of the clinic.

Most instruments comprise a probe, which may be hermetically sealed in the ear canal using a small plastic cuff or probe tip. Within the probe are three components (Figure 6.1). A miniature earphone provides the sound source which is a pure tone (usually at 226 Hz); this is delivered to the ear by a flexible tube within the probe. A miniature microphone is also joined to the probe via a flexible tube; this measures the sound pressure level (SPL) within the ear canal. An air pump connected to a manometer indicates the air pressure in the ear canal relative to atmospheric pressure. Manometers of older instruments are

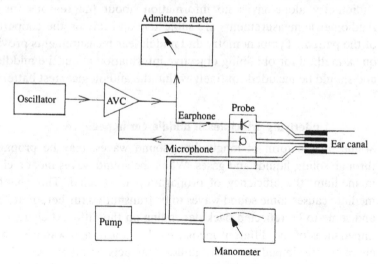

Figure 6.1. Block diagram of a middle-ear measurement system (AVC = automatic volume control).

calibrated in millimetres of water pressure (mmH_2O) and more recent instruments are calibrated in the SI units of decapascal (daPa); however this is really only of academic interest as the two units are virtually equivalent (1 daPa = 1.02 mmH_2O).

Terminology

Admittance: This is a measure of how efficiently the tympanic membrane and middle-ear system receive and transmit sound energy travelling down the ear canal. (In reality it is the sum of ear canal admittance and middle ear admittance.)

Compliance: Most clinical instruments express admittance in terms of compliance. Strictly this is a misnomer, as compliance is only one of the components of admittance, however under the test conditions used and with a low frequency probe tone, it is a reasonable approximation.

Impedance: This is the reciprocal of admittance.

Immitance: This is a generic term incorporating acoustic impedance and admittance.

Tympanometry

This is perhaps the most commonly used measurement of middle-ear measurement systems. The output of the probe microphone is used to control the sound level by an automatic volume (gain) control (Figure 6.1). Keeping the SPL constant enables the admittance modulator at the end of the probe to measure the driving force needed to maintain this constant SPL within the ear canal. Thus, for an ear with high admittance, a large driving force is required, and for an ear with low admittance a small driving force is required. A highly mobile ear will produce a high admittance to incoming sound, and an immobile ear will produce a low admittance.

Most pathological conditions of the middle ear alter the way the tympanic membrane reacts to acoustical energy and adversely affect the elasticity and hence the mobility of the middle-ear system. Some also affect the mass of the system. Middle-ear effusion loads the inner surface of the tympanic membrane and middle ear as well as stiffening the membrane. Thus admittance measurements can provide useful diagnostic indications about the state of the middle ear.

The middle-ear measurement system may be manually or automatically operated. To measure a tympanogram, the air pressure is varied within the ear canal (usually from +200 to –200 daPa) and the equivalent air volume is measured. A graphic printout is produced of admittance, as equivalent air volume, against pressure: this is the tympanogram. The two most commonly used measurements taken from the tympanogram are those of middle-ear pressure and middle-ear compliance. The volume of the ear canal can also be estimated.

Middle-ear pressure (MEP)

In general, as the air pressure in the ear canal is progressively increased or decreased with respect to the MEP by use of the air pump, the tympanic membrane becomes increasingly inflexible and the compliance decreases. Maximum compliance is found at the point where air pressure in the ear canal and middle-ear pressure are equal. This is the point of MEP relative to atmospheric pressure. Normal MEP ranges from +50 to –100 daPa.

Middle-ear compliance (MEC)

When the air pressure in the ear canal is at MEP, the compliance is that of the air in the ear canal and the middle-ear structures. As the air pressure in the ear canal is progressively increased or decreased, the compliance of the tympanic membrane and middle ear becomes increasingly smaller to a point where compliance is approximately equal to that of the air in the ear canal. The difference between this value and that of maximum compliance is approximately equal to MEC. Normal MEC ranges from 0.3 to 1.5 cm^3.

Middle-ear volume

The compliance at each end of the tympanogram (where compliance is lowest) approximates to middle-ear volume (cm^3).

Interpretation of the tympanogram and pathological conditions

Low compliance values

Otosclerosis, fibrosis and tympanosclerosis are all conditions which cause a stiffening or reduction in movement of the tympanic membrane. This gives a tympanogram indicating reduced compliance at normal pressure (curve (a) in Figure 6.2). It should, however, be remembered that there is a large range of normal compliance values and the value of the tympanograms in diagnosing the above conditions is often questioned. As with all the middle-ear measurement test results, this type of tympanogram is of most use when considered in conjunction with other audiometric test results and a good medical history.

High compliance values

Ossicular discontinuity often gives rise to high compliance values (curve (b) Figure 6.2); however a thinning of the tympanic membrane may give a similar result indicating hypermobility. Again it is important to consider the large range of normal values.

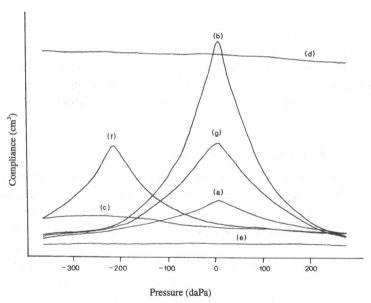

Figure 6.2. Example of some typical tympanograms: (a) otosclerosis, (b) hypermobility, (c) middle-ear effusions, (d) perforated tympanic membrane, (e) blocked ear canal or probe, (f) Eustachian tube dysfunction, (g) normal tympanogram.

Flat tympanograms

Tympanograms are probably of most diagnostic use and are usually indicative of middle-ear effusion (curve (c) Figure 6.2). This is therefore probably the most common type of tympanogram encountered in paediatric audiology. Middle-ear effusion causes a loading of the whole middle-ear system, which in turn causes the tympanic membranes to stiffen. Middle-ear conditions give rise to a shallow or virtually flat tympanogram with reduced compliance and pressure. Other pathological conditions can cause stiffness of the tympanic membrane but in children, this result usually indicates the presence of middle ear effusions.

High middle-ear volume

This result is often indicative of a perforated tympanic membrane. The flat 'curve' (curve (d) Figure 6.2) represents the combined volume of the ear canal and middle-ear cavity. A similar result may indicate a patent grommet. A very high middle-ear volume may be an indication that the probe was not sealed properly in the ear canal.

Low middle-ear volume

A flat 'curve' with a middle-ear volume close to zero (curve (e) Figure 6.2) is often an indication of a blocked ear canal, frequently due to wax occlusion. This result may also be obtained if the probe is being held against the wall of the ear canal or if the probe is itself blocked.

Low MEP with normal MEC

This result is often an indication of Eustachian tube dysfunction (curve (f) Figure 6.2). Occasionally autoinflation with a 'sticky' Eustachian tube may give a result of positive middle-ear pressure. If the subject performs a successful Valsalva or Toynbee manoeuvre the tympanogram may change indicating an increase in MEP. A flat tympanogram may indicate the presence of middle-ear fluid in conjunction with Eustachian tube dysfunction; however it may be that the viscosity of the fluid makes its removal from the middle-ear impossible even in the presence of normal Eustachian tube function. An unusual possibility is that of a patent Eustachian tube, which sometimes follows persistent middle-ear effusion. This may give rise to the pressure meter indicating rising and falling pressure in time with respiration and sub-jects may experience an 'echo' as they speak. Similar variations in pressure may be observed in some normal ears.

A *normal tympanogram*

As has already been mentioned, most pathological conditions of the middle ear affect the tympanogram; therefore a normal tympanogram (curve (g) Figure 6.2) is a fairly good indication of normal middle-ear function.

Pitfalls in measurement and interpretation of the tympanogram

The tympanogram is an invaluable measure of middle-ear function with a high sensitivity and specificity for indicating pathological states, but it is not completely infallible. It is imperative that the tympanometric measurements are not considered in isolation but are viewed as part of an audiological test battery. Failure to do this may lead to misdiagnosis and hence mismanagement.

Sources of error may relate to the measurement process itself. Particularly during the testing of children and infants it may be that the subject moves during the measurement, or may be particularly noisy. These two events may cause movement of the probe causing misleading peaks to appear on the tympanogram. In this case the tympanogram should be repeated where possible or an appropriate note should be attached to the tympanogram and the interpretation made with caution.

Another possible complication is that there may be more than one condition present. Sensorineural hearing loss alone will give rise to a normal tympanogram. The sensorineural hearing loss may, however, be present in conjunction with middle-ear effusion. In cases where a flat tympanogram is present in conjunction with a hearing loss, particularly where the loss is moderate, severe or profound, the tests of hearing and middle-ear measurements should be repeated on later occasions until a sensorineural hearing loss can be eliminated. Failure to test the hearing in conjunction with performing the tympanogram, or assuming the hearing loss is purely conductive, can lead to missing a diagnosis of sensorineural hearing loss and hence delayed intervention. Finally, there is a large range of normal test results and hence some pathological conditions may not be apparent. In addition some normal ears may give abnormal results on a tympanogram for reasons which are not clear.

Diagnostic errors may be avoided by considering tympanometric results in conjunction with a detailed history and other audiological test results and by ensuring that the person undertaking the testing is well trained.

Middle-ear stapedial reflex measurements

Stapedial reflex measurements can usually be carried out using the same middle-ear measurement equipment. When a normal ear is stimulated with a 'loud' sound, the stapedius muscle in both middle ears contracts, causing a stiffening of the tympanic membranes and hence a decrease in compliance. This compliance change can be detected by the middle-ear measurement system already described. This reflex measurement is of use diagnostically.

Acoustic reflex threshold (ART)

Normal ears have a reflex threshold of 80 to 85 dBHL for pure tone frequencies between 250 and 4000 Hz. A screening test may use a mid-frequency tone at 90 to 100 dBHL. Presence of a reflex at this level indicates that the middle ear is free from significant disorder.

In cases of normal hearing the ART is approximately 85 dB above the hearing threshold but in cases of sensorineural hearing loss, the ART is often far closer to the hearing threshold. In cases where the difference between ART and hearing threshold is 65 dB or less, this may indicate the presence of abnormal loudness function (recruitment). In some cases of sensorineural hearing loss the ART will be higher than the limits of the middle-ear measurement system and in such cases it is important to consider the results of this test in conjunction with other middle-ear and audiological test results to determine whether absence of the acoustic reflex is due to a conductive or sensorineural hearing loss.

Acoustic reflex decay (ARD)

Acoustic reflex decay is another measurement of diagnostic value. This test is undertaken by stimulating the ear with a tone 10 dB above the ART. In a normal ear, the stapedius will contract for the duration of the stimulus within a time span of a few minutes; the usual duration of stimulus on this test is 10 seconds. The amount of ARD is measured as the percentage reduction in compliance during the 10 seconds. Greater than 50% decay in 5 seconds is thought to be diagnostically significant in terms of VIII nerve pathology. Acoustic reflex tests are of far greater diagnostic value when they are considered in conjunction with each other and with the tympanometric results.

Middle-ear effusion

Middle-ear effusion is well known to be the most common cause of auditory dysfunction in children. It is, in fact, so common that it could be thought to be part of normal development. In most cases of middle-ear effusion there is little cause for concern; however for a few children, this condition does give rise to long term problems. Problems tend to arise with children who have persistent middle-ear effusion, who may display difficulties such as behavioural problems and even developmental delay in some cases. This condition can be treated using medical, surgical or audiological intervention; however the time at which this is most effective, or indeed whether it is actually needed, is a matter for some debate. Parent and teacher counselling and advice is often of great value in these cases.

Middle-ear measurements offer a simple screening test for middle-ear effusion. There are, however, several drawbacks to this. Firstly, since it is such a common condition, tympanometry and middle-ear measurements, in the absence of audiometry or behavioural hearing tests, will pick up too many cases to be manageable and far more cases than need active intervention. Many children will give a flat tympanogram for a short time, which is of no consequence during episodes of upper respiratory tract infections. The cases of middle-ear effusion most in need of treatment are those that are persistent. In order to find these cases it is necessary to carry out testing at intervals over a period of time. Secondly, it is not only the middle-ear measurements or tympanogram that should be considered when deciding on possible intervention; degree of hearing loss and degree of disability to the child need also to be considered. Therefore, any 'screening' for middle-ear effusion or otitis media with effusion should be carried out by appropriately trained professionals and the middle-ear measurements should be just one of the considerations taken into account when considering management.

Further reading

Beery, Q. C., Bluestone, C. D., Andrus, W. S. and Cantekin, E. (1975). Tympanometry pattern classification in relation to middle ear effusions. *Annals of Otology, Rhinology and Laryngology*, **84**, 56–64.

Brooks, D. N. (1969). The use of the electroacoustical impedance bridge in the assessment of middle ear function. *International Audiology*, **8**, 563–9.

Brooks, D. N. (1988). Acoustic measurement of auditory function. In *Paediatric Audiology 0–5 years*, 2nd edn, (ed. B. McCormick). London: Whurr Publishers Limited.

Jerger, J., Jerger, S. and Mouldin, L. (1972). Studies in impedance audiometry I: Normal and sensorineural ears. *Archives of Otolaryngology*, **96**, 513–23.

Paradise, J. L., Smith, C. G. and Bluestone, C. D. (1976). Tympanometric detection of middle ear effusion in infants and young children. *Pediatrics*, **58**, 198–210.

Shallop, J. K. (1976). The historical development of the study of middle ear function. In *Acoustical Impedance and Admittance – the Measurement of Middle Ear Function* (ed. A. S. Feldman and L. A. Wilber), pp. 8–48. Baltimore: Williams and Wilkins.

7

The management of otitis media with effusion

NICK JONES and SUSAN ROBINSON

Scope of the chapter

Otitis media with effusion is the most common cause of hearing impairment and reason for elective surgery in children. In most cases no specific treatment is required and the important role of the medical practitioner is to identify the small number of cases that warrant treatment or onward referral. This chapter aims to provide background information on the condition and a practical guide to assist medical practitioners in this task.

Introduction

Otitis media with effusion (OME) is a normal finding in children following an upper respiratory tract infection and the majority of OME resolves spontaneously. Only a small minority of approximately 4.7 per 1000 children come to surgery in Britain. While many have focused their attention on the appearance of the drum or tympanometric tracing, *it is the history that is all-important in the management of OME.*

Hearing screening attempts to identify children whose hearing loss is sufficient to affect their language and speech development. It is of primary importance to ensure that children with a sensorineural hearing loss are not missed, and every effort should be made to try and find these children as early as possible, although logistically this is difficult. This group has to be differentiated from the large number of children with OME. Many children will need following up as a result of screening. The system varies from district to district depending on the resources available but follow-up may be undertaken by a variety of staff. In addition to children seen as a result of screening the medical practitioner will also see those brought to the surgery by concerned parents.

The medical practitioner's role

It is essential to discuss with parents the nature of OME, what the treatment options are, the potential consequences of OME, and the natural history of the condition. This avoids 'medicalising' what is most frequently a natural process that will resolve on its own. The decision as to whether one should wait for resolution or intervene, is based on how the child is functioning and where in the natural history of OME the child is thought to be. For example, in a young child who is asymptomatic and whose language is developing well, the need to intervene in OME is reduced.

The sequelae of untreated OME should also be considered. Not only are there short and medium term problems caused by hearing loss, pain from recurrent acute otitis media and sometimes from even mild Eustachian tube dysfunction, but persistently low middle-ear pressure can cause thinning of the drum (atelectasis), retraction and resorption of the ossicular chain with long term effects.

The question, 'Who is helped by surgery?' is difficult to answer specifically as *the effects of OME are not all-or-none. Treatment, whether conservative or surgical, should be undertaken in the light of the child's language and general development, and the length of the history.* In this chapter we aim to guide the medical practitioner through the various stages in the management of this condition.

Classification of otitis media

Acute otitis media (AOM)

Acute otitis media (AOM) is characterised by pain, a raised temperature and earache. Initially the eardrum is red and if enough purulent fluid is produced it may bulge and eventually perforate with a purulent discharge, but with cessation of pain. The majority of children with AOM have a viral infection which resolves within 24 hours of onset. Symptoms which persist after 24 hours from onset are more likely to be bacterial and warrant antibiotic treatment.

Recurrent AOM

Recurrent episodes each with a 15% incidence of subsequent OME.

Otitis media with effusion (OME)

Otitis media with effusion is generally characterised by a persistent accumulation of non-purulent and mucoid fluid in the middle ear. This leads to a dull and opaque appearance to the eardrum. It also restricts movement of the eardrum and ossicles and in some cases results in a hearing loss. Whilst the middle-ear fluid contains pathogens in approximately 17% of patients, they are not in sufficient numbers for the fluid to be considered infected.

Chronic suppurative otitis media

This term is usually applied to an ear that discharges mucus through a perforated eardrum.

1. Safe or tubotympanic disease: a perforation in the pars tensa or lower nine-tenths of the ear-drum. (Safe perforations form the vast majority of tympanic perforations. Whilst cholesteatoma is rare in this group it nevertheless is a possibility and should not be excluded.)
2. Unsafe or attico-antral disease: a defect in the attic area associated with cholesteatoma.

Prevalence and natural history of OME

The incidence (new cases) of OME is greatest in the 6 to 12 month age group with 75–80% of that age group having one or more episodes. Around 42% of 3-year-olds may begin an episode of OME over the next 12 months. Because each episode is generally of short duration the percentage of children with OME at any one time (prevalence) is much lower. There is a peak of approximately 20% around 2 years of age and a second peak of approximately 15% around 5 years of age. Prevalence of OME falls off sharply between the ages of 6 and 8 to less than 5%.

Whilst OME is extremely common, the vast majority of cases resolve naturally. For example, in over 50% of affected 2-year-olds it resolves spontaneously within 3 months and only 3% of them will have an episode lasting over one year. However, a further 9% will have had one or more recurrences by the time they are 3 years old.

The main risk factors for OME include age, sex (more common in boys than girls), season (more occur in winter), bottle feeding, attendance at day care and passive smoking. Anatomical abnormalities of the face such as cleft palate, reduced postnasal space and certain genetic syndromes (e.g. Down's, Turner's, Hunter's, fragile X) and abnormalities of the skull base and nasopharynx are also associated with an increased risk of persistent OME.

Hearing impairment and disability

Only a minority of those with OME have a material hearing loss. The impairment is conductive, commonly fluctuating and typically 20–30 dBHL in magnitude. At any point in time about 6% of children aged 2 years (i.e. approximately one-third of those with OME) will have a bilateral hearing impairment in excess of 25 dBHL persisting for 3 months or more.

A number of disabilities may result from persistent hearing impairment (e.g. compromised levels of social functioning, language competence and speech production, learning or behavioural difficulties). Studies that have examined the consequences of persistent OME have failed to demonstrate a significant and causal link.

The lack of a consistent relationship does not negate the fact that OME can lead to material disability. This may be due to interaction with other factors such as family circumstances, intelligence, general health and other disabilities. Therefore identification of persistent cases (e.g. hearing impairment lasting more than 6 months) is recommended. These will include those cases at risk of disability and therefore most likely to benefit from intervention.

History

The aim is to assess the extent and persistence of any hearing loss based on the parent's description of everyday situations. The following questions may be used as a guide:

1. Have parents, teachers or carers noticed any hearing difficulties? If so, for how long?
2. Does the child's hearing appear to fluctuate?
3. Is language developing normally? Has the expected milestone been reached?
4. Have there been any changes in the child's behaviour patterns?
5. Has there been frequent upper respiratory tract infection?

6. How many episodes of AOM have there been (earache, discharge, etc.)?

Multiple episodes are less likely to be associated with the resolution of any middle-ear effusion. It is worth trying to establish if these were genuine episodes of AOM or not; severe pain followed by discharge is diagnostic, while pyrexia and earache that is short lived, are not.

The history should include any other relevant factors that might predispose to OME (e.g. Down's syndrome, cleft palate) and other disabilities including a pre-existing sensorineural hearing loss, family circumstances and developmental delay. It is useful to ask about permanent hearing impairment in order that a sensorineural hearing loss is not missed. Additionally, questions relating to other otological pathology are relevant (e.g. a foul discharging ear means that cholesteatoma should be excluded). Other developmental milestones should be noted to ensure that there is not a global problem that requires further investigation.

Examination

A general examination should be done looking for any abnormal features of the face and skull, any features of genetic syndromes, mouth breathing and/or voice quality (i.e. hyponasality). In an acute episode it is important to look behind the ear, particularly to exclude mastoiditis. For inspection of the external ear canal, the pinna should be pulled back gently and firmly to straighten the ear canal. It may be very narrow in children with Down's syndrome and in neonates, and it is liable to collapse in young children. Using an otoscope is made easier if the (young) child is appropriately restrained, usually by the parent, as shown in Figure 7.1.

It is important to inspect the eardrum using an otoscope in order to help define whether any hearing loss can be explained by OME or whether there may be some other pathology. The otoscope should be held using one of the fingers of the hand resting on the child to detect early movement that the child might make and prevent the instrument traumatising the ear canal (see Figure 7.2). Features of OME at the eardrum include a dull appearance, the absence of light reflex, increased vascularity of the drum, a more horizontal position of the malleus handle and retraction of the drum. If there are air bubbles or a fluid level with clear fluid, this is a sign of resolving OME. Other

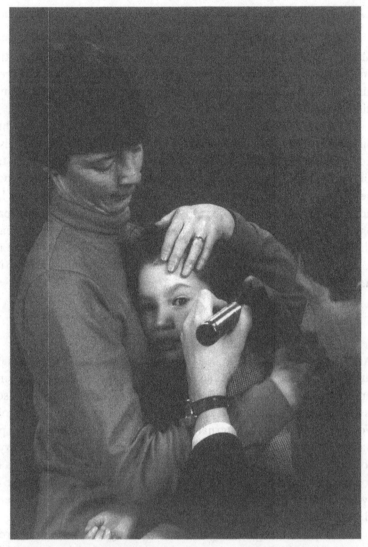

Figure 7.1. Examination of the ear – the child may need to be restrained.

middle-ear pathologies, particularly a perforation of the drum or a cholesteatoma, need to be excluded whilst examining the ear. It is frequently difficult to be certain whether there is glue from the otoscopic appearance alone. It is not the appearance of the ear-drum on any particular day that is important but how the child is functioning.

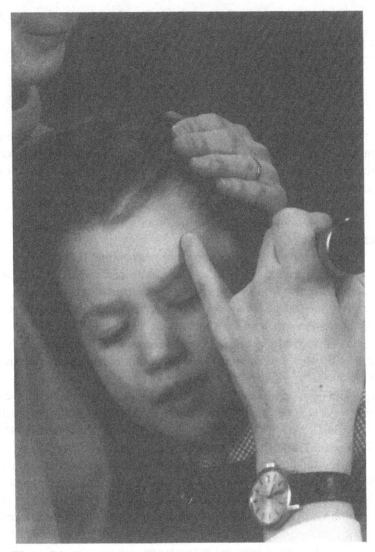

Figure 7.2. Examination of the ear – the examiner's little finger rests on the child.

Pointers to the presence of other middle-ear pathology include:

1. A crust in the attic area may hide an underlying cholesteatoma.
2. Congenital cholesteatoma is rare but should be looked for. It has the appearance of a white pearl behind the drum.

3. A mucoid discharge implies that there is a perforation as the external ear canal has no mucus glands.
4. A foul discharge should raise the question of an underlying cholesteatoma.

Wax

Wax often obstructs the view. Wax in the external third of the canal may be removed with little difficulty – it is unwise for anyone without the experience or the equipment to delve deeper. It is unusual for there to be any justification for the immediate removal of wax. It is far more important to make some assessment of how the child is functioning than to remove wax in order to view the drum and diagnose the presence of effusion.

The best tools to remove wax from the external half of the ear canal are either a wax hook or a Jobson Horne probe, using the light of a headmirror. It is important to avoid causing any discomfort and if there is any difficulty removing the wax it is far better to prescribe sodium bicarbonate eardrops (8%) twice daily to dissolve the wax and then review the child's progress. Otoscopes with a distal fibreoptic light source provide a far superior view of the drum. Most modern otoscopes have an attachment for a rubber bulb for pneumatic otoscopy – if a speculum can be inserted that will seal off the ear canal the bulb can be gently pressed and the mobility of the drum inspected – with practice it is possible to see if the mobility is reduced (indicating Eustachian tube dysfunction) or absent as in OME.

During the otoscopic examination, it is useful in older children (over 5 years) to conduct a clinical hearing test such as asking a question in a quiet voice. As they will not see you speaking, this may give an opportunity broadly to assess the extent of their hearing difficulties and find out if there may be a non-organic hearing loss. The following observations should also be included in the examination:

1. Is the child mouth breathing?
2. Does the child speak with a hyponasal voice?
3. Does the child have a nasal crease?

Nasal obstruction in children is usually due to allergic rhinitis, adenoidal hypertrophy and infection, either on their own or together.

Ask whether the child *persistently* mouth breathes, snores or has a 'snotty nose'. Children average eight upper respiratory tract infections a year and therefore it is not unusual for a child to have a snotty nose intermittently for many months. Ask when the child last had a clear nose; if it was less than 4 months ago it makes it unlikely that adenoidal hypertrophy is a significant factor. Perennial symptoms may be due to an allergy to house dust mite. This is often overlooked as a cause for nasal obstruction. The role of allergic rhinitis in OME is controversial. In 2–5-year-olds adenoidal hypertrophy is associated with recurrence of OME following grommet extrusion.

Hearing assessment

Few medical practices will have the facilities and personnel to carry out accurate quantitative tests of hearing and middle-ear function (e.g. sufficiently low and verified ambient noise levels, calibrated equipment, suitably trained personnel). The role of the medical practitioner is to assess the child's disability as perceived by carers and to make an informal assessment of hearing ability. This information will help to decide which children require referral for formal hearing assessment, based on persistence of symptoms and risk factors. The formal assessment of hearing will include measurements of hearing sensitivity, tympanometric measures of middle-ear function and determination of whether the hearing loss is sensorineural or conductive. For details of tests and their interpretation see Chapters 3, 4, 5 and 6. Tympanometry provides confirmative evidence of OME but it should not detract from the primary consideration of how the child is functioning in terms of language and hearing.

Management in general practice

Because of the characteristics of this condition, in which a significant proportion of children recover spontaneously, there is justifiable uncertainty as to when referral or treatment is appropriate. We advocate a period of '*watchful waiting*', where the child is monitored to establish that the condition is persistent. Reassurance should be given to the family regarding the nature and cause of the child's condition. Advice on compensating tactics should be provided. The following compensation tactics may be useful:

1. Speak close to the child so that the level of voice is slightly raised, but do not shout.

2. Speak clearly but do not exaggerate mouth movements.
3. Face the child so that the speaker can be seen and heard.
4. Try to reduce background noise when communicating with the child, e.g. switch off or turn down the television.
5. Inform all family members, carers, teachers or playgroup leaders and friends about the child's hearing difficulties and explain how they can help.

Antibiotics do not have a convincing therapeutic effect on OME. Similarly there is no evidence that decongestants alter the condition. Anti-allergy treatment – avoiding aggravating allergens, the use of anti-histamines and topical nasal steroids (fluticasone is licensed for use in 4-year-olds) – will help nasal symptoms resulting from allergic rhinitis and may improve Eustachian tube function in atopic children.

At the end of the period of observation (e.g. 3 months) the child must be reviewed to establish the need for referral using the criteria of persistence and disability. Further otoscopy should be undertaken to ensure that no other middle-ear pathology is present. Progressive retraction of the drum with ossicular erosion, deepening of a retraction pocket, or the drum becoming adherent to the medial wall of the middle ear warrants early referral for an otological opinion.

Management following a period of 'watchful waiting'

Having introduced a period of 'watchful waiting', the group of children eventually treated will be those more likely to benefit from surgery. Grommet insertion reduces the mean hearing impairment in children with OME. Myringotomy alone is not effective in restoring hearing levels. There is no added benefit of tonsillectomy in the treatment of OME. Grommets temporarily improve hearing when in place and functioning. The effect of treatment diminishes with time. The mean improvement in hearing is estimated to be less than 12 dBHL at 6 months and under 6 dBHL at 12 months. The clinical significance of this improvement is not clear. Adenoidectomy may have a role in 2–5-year-olds with persistent OME who undergo grommet insertion; it appears to reduce the likelihood of requiring further grommets.

Hearing aids also restore hearing levels in cases of persistent conductive hearing loss although adaptation to using these may pose a problem (see Chapter 9). This option is particularly suitable for cases where surgery is contraindicated or OME is a recurrent problem (e.g. children with Down's syndrome or cleft palate; repeated early extrusion of grommets; persistent discharge through a grommet, in spite of topical antibiotic eardrops; or when parents decline surgery).

Advice and specific support should also be available to both parents and teachers during the 'watchful waiting' period and treatment or monitoring stages. This may be supplemented by written guidelines. This stage in the management of OME is essential, as the aim of 'watchful waiting' is to delay the decision to operate until need has been fully established using criteria such as persistence and severity. The subset of children eventually treated may wait longer and therefore may experience an extended period of hearing impairment. Schedules for follow-

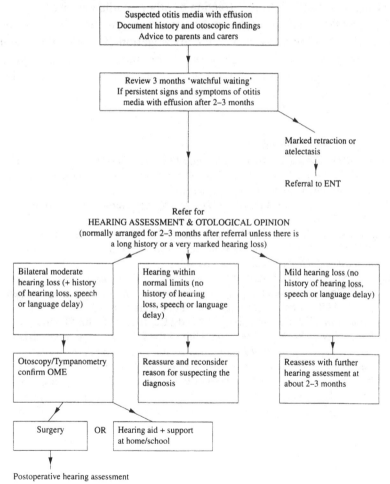

Figure 7.3. The management of otitis media with effusion.

up, which will include further hearing and middle-ear assessment, are given in Figure 7.3.

Summary

Otitis media with effusion is extremely common in children. The medical practitioner has the task of sorting out from this large group the children who have persistent OME, which will affect their development. OME resolves spontaneously in the majority of children and so 'watchful waiting' is usually the best initial course, unless there are features that cause concern such as possible moderate or severe sensorineural hearing loss, marked drum retraction or other middle-ear disease.

When OME fails to resolve and there is concern about hearing, well conducted hearing assessment is the investigation of choice. Treatment, whether conservative or surgical, should be undertaken in the light of the child's language and general development, and the length of the history of OME.

Further reading

Anon (1987). *Making the Most of Hearing: Ideas to help children who have a mild conductive loss*. Bristol: Avon Services for Special Educational Needs and Southmead Speech Therapy Service.

Chole, R. A. (1982). *An Atlas of Ear Disease*. Weert, Netherlands: Wolfe Medical.

Haggard, M. P., Gannon, M. M. and Spencer, H. (1992). The paediatric otological caseload resulting from improved screening in the first year of life. *Clinical Otolaryngology*, **17**, 34–43.

Haggard, M. P., Birkin, J. A. and Pringle, D. P. (1993). Consequences of otitis media for speech and language. In *Paediatric Audiology 0–5 years*, 2nd edn (ed. B. McCormick). London: Whurr Publishers Limited.

School of Public Health, University of Leeds, Centre for Health Economics, University of York and Research Unit of the Royal College of Physicians (1992). *The Treatment of Persistent Glue Ear in Children: Are Surgical Interventions Effective in Combating Disability From Glue Ear*. Effective Health Care No. 4. Leeds: School of Public Health, University of Leeds.

Stephenson, H. and Haggard, M. P. (1992). Rationale and design of surgical trials for Otitis Media with Effusion. *Clinical Otolaryngology*, **17**, 67–78.

8

Management of unilateral hearing loss

SALLY WOOD

Introduction

Unilateral hearing loss occurs when there is some degree of hearing loss in one ear with normal hearing in the other. Many children suffer from conductive hearing loss in childhood and some of these may be unilateral losses for some of the time. This chapter, however, is concerned with the case of permanent unilateral loss, which is almost always sensorineural in nature.

Prevalence

Accurate figures for the presence of unilateral sensorineural loss are hard to come by. Some studies (Everberg, 1960; Tarkkanen and Aho, 1966) have estimated prevalence at around 1 : 1000 in school children.

Aetiology

Aetiological information is also problematic and the well known difficulties in establishing aetiology for sensorineural hearing loss are compounded in the case of unilateral loss by the often relatively late age at which it is ascertained. Many studies have suggested that unknown aetiology is the largest group (approximately 50%) with mumps, measles and meningitis accounting for the majority of identifiable causes.

Psychoacoustic advantages of binaural hearing

There are several advantages to binaural hearing and it follows that the unilaterally impaired child is deprived of these. The main psychoacoustic phenomena related to binaural hearing are as follows.

Binaural summation: The binaural threshold is around 3 dB better than the monaural threshold. This also applies to supra-threshold stimuli so that binaural sounds are louder than monaural sounds by between 3 and 6 dB.

Localisation: For a given sound source there are time and intensity differences between the signals arriving at the two ears and these are used as cues to localisation. This ability is impaired in unilaterally hearing-impaired subjects (Bess, 1982; Newton, 1983).

Head shadow effects: This refers to the acoustic shadow of the head. Its effect is that acoustic signals coming from the right side are louder in the right ear than the left ear and vice versa. The higher the frequency the more pronounced the effect since lower frequency sounds are better able to 'bend' around the head and reach the contralateral ear.

Precedence effect: This is the effect by which sounds reaching the ear in close succession are heard as a single sound. It is particularly important when listening in reverberant environments and is essentially a binaural phenomenon (Moore, 1989).

Squelch effect: When speech and noise are presented at the same time but are spatially separated there is an improvement in speech discrimination in the case of binaural listening compared with monaural listening.

In general, binaural processing contributes to the ability to localise sounds and also to the ability to detect and analyse signals in noisy and reverberant conditions. Unfortunately these are just the sort of conditions that often prevail in educational settings and in everyday listening situations.

Effects of unilateral hearing loss

The extent to which unilateral losses result in educational, linguistic or cognitive difficulties for the child is debatable and the evidence is unclear. Some studies (Hallmo *et al.*, 1986) have shown few educational or communication problems whereas others (Bess and Tharpe, 1986; Hartvig Jensen *et al.*, 1989 a, b) have suggested an increased risk of educational problems especially for right-ear impaired children. Colletti *et al.* (1988) looked at a group of adults who had suffered unilateral hearing loss since childhood and found no evidence to support the existence of non-auditory long term effects although they again demonstrated the superiority of binaural compared with monaural hearing.

Assessment of unilateral hearing loss

Assessment of hearing levels is carried out using the techniques described in Chapters 3–6. The main difficulty arises in the measurement of accurate thresholds for the worse hearing ear. Sound field tests generally reflect the status of the better hearing ear and although they can often point to the existence of a degree of unilateral loss it is not usually possible to assess the poorer ear thresholds accurately, particularly when the better ear is normal. In order to assess the poor ear hearing levels accurately pure tone audiometry with masking as described in Chapter 4 is necessary. The child may therefore be 4 or 5 years old before it is possible to measure accurately the worse ear hearing levels. All children with unilateral hearing loss should be seen by a consultant otolaryngologist. There are numerous pathologies that can give rise to progressive unilateral sensorineural hearing loss and although extremely rare in children these need to be considered.

Parents are often quite shocked and upset to find that their child has a severe or profound unilateral hearing loss, particularly as they have often not previously suspected any hearing difficulties. It is important to reassure them that this is often the case with such children and that it is unlikely that an earlier diagnosis would have conferred any great advantage.

Management of unilateral hearing loss

Once the otological and audiological assessment has been completed, the main focus in the management of this condition is on appropriate advice and guidance on hearing tactics and the assessment of the need for amplification. It is important to ensure that parents, friends, relatives and teachers are aware of the existence of the hearing loss and its possible effects. The use of written information and leaflets is often extremely helpful. It is important to explain that whilst the child may have few obvious difficulties with speech discrimination in quiet there are likely to be specific difficulties with the following:

detecting sound or hearing speech on the poor side
hearing speech in noise
locating the source of sound

Hearing tactics

If at all possible one should avoid addressing speech directly to the side
of the poor ear, particularly when there is a lot of background noise.
This is not always possible, particularly in group situations, and it may
be necessary to attract the child's attention before addressing him/her.
Similarly in noisy situations we all benefit from visual cues to some
extent and this will also be important for the child with unilateral hearing loss.

Classroom seating

Teachers in particular need to be aware of the nature and degree of the
hearing loss and of the importance of strategies such as preferential

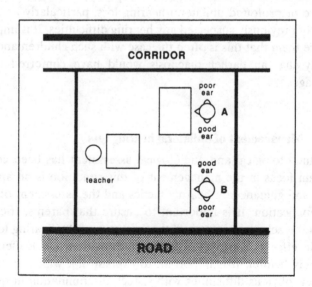

Figure 8.1. Good seating arrangements in a conventional classroom.

seating arrangements. The child should be seated so that he/she can see the teacher and with the good ear directed towards the teacher. The poor ear, wherever possible, should be directed towards any potential source of unwanted noise, for example a corridor or traffic. The child should be seated as near to the teacher as possible. Figure 8.1 shows a sensible seating arrangement for child A (with a right-sided hearing loss) and child B (with a left-sided hearing loss) in a conventional class-room. Figure 8.2 shows the same children in the same classroom but this time with poor seating arrangements. Many children, particularly young children, are not taught in such formally arranged classrooms. In these cases it is even more important that the teacher is aware of the hearing loss and is able to be flexible in the seating arrangements. Figure 8.3 shows a good seating arrangement for a child with a right-sided hearing loss and Figure 8.4 shows examples of poor seating for the same child.

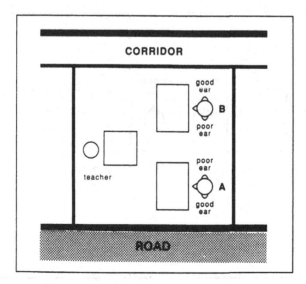

Figure 8.2. Poor seating arrangements in a conventional classroom.

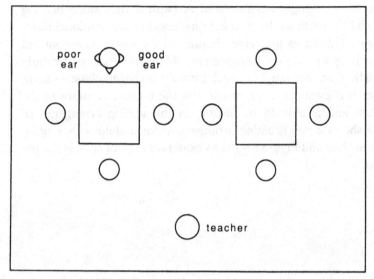

Figure 8.3. Good seating arrangements in a group situation.

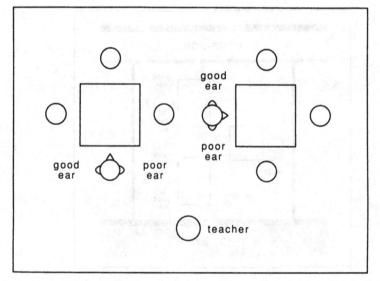

Figure 8.4. Poor seating arrangements in a group situation.

Road safety

Children with unilateral hearing loss will probably have impaired localisation ability and therefore they may not be able to locate and react to warning signals, for example a car horn, very quickly. The child needs to be given careful road safety instruction and special precautions taken, for example fitting and use of bicycle mirrors are advisable.

Amplification

The benefit from a conventional hearing aid is likely to be very limited for children with unilateral losses. In the case of a mild or moderate loss there may be some benefit from an aid in particular situations but this is likely to be highly variable between individuals. For more severe losses the use of a conventional powerful aid, which would be required to provide sufficient amplification to the poor ear, is contraindicated. In such a case a CROS aid may be helpful in certain situations. CROS is an acronym for Contralateral Routing Of Signals and involves wearing a hearing aid microphone on the poor ear to pick up the auditory signal and then routing this into the good ear by means of a hard wire or a radio link. Successful use of this device requires a considerable amount of sophistication and motivation on the part of the child.

Some workers (Bess and Tharpe, 1986) are suggesting that for a child who is experiencing difficulty in the educational setting the most appropriate form of amplification is an FM or radio system used in conjunction with a low power hearing aid in the good ear as a means to improve the signal-to-noise ratio. This would require extremely careful setting up and use in order to ensure that it is used consistently and appropriately in the classroom and that the child is not subject to unduly high output levels with consequent risk to hearing sensitivity in the good ear.

Parents may ask about cochlear implants, which are sometimes portrayed in the media as a 'cure' for deafness. They need to be advised that these are not appropriate for unilateral hearing loss (see Chapter 10).

Hearing conservation

Parents need to be given advice about audiological and otological care. This includes the following:

to seek prompt medical advice and treatment for any otological problems, particularly in the good ear. A child who is dependent upon the hearing in one ear will be significantly disadvantaged by any temporary hearing loss in that ear associated with middle-ear problems;

to seek reassessment of the child's hearing if there are any signs of change in the hearing levels;

to avoid placing or poking objects into the ear canal;

to avoid prolonged exposure to very loud noise, for example loud rock concerts or personal stereos on high volume settings; the use of appropriate ear protection later in life if this is required because of a noisy occupation or noisy hobby (for example, shooting).

Summary

Children with unilateral hearing loss are often diagnosed relatively late on and the confirmation often comes as a considerable shock to parents who have not previously suspected any hearing difficulties. The aetiology of the hearing loss is often difficult to ascertain with any certainty, particularly in the absence of any obvious causative factors such as measles, mumps or meningitis. Most children with unilateral hearing loss cope extremely well but they do face a number of hearing difficulties resulting from the loss of binaural processing. It is very important that all those involved with the child, particularly in the educational context, are aware of the nature of the hearing difficulties experienced. The use of written information leaflets or booklets is often very helpful.

References

Bess, F. H. (1982). Children with unilateral hearing loss. *Journal of the Academy of Rehabilitative Audiology*, **15**, 131–44.

Bess, F. H. and Tharpe, A. M. (ed.) (1986). Unilateral sensorineural hearing loss in children. *Ear and Hearing*, **7**, 2–54.

Colletti, V., Fiorino, F. G., Carner, M. and Rizzi, R. (1988). Investigation of the long-term effects of unilateral hearing loss in adults. *British Journal of Audiology*, **22**, 113–18.

Everberg, G. (1960). Etiology of unilateral total deafness studied in a series of children and young adults. *Annals of Otology, Rhinology and Laryngology*, **69**, 711–30.

Hallmo, P., Moller, P., Lind, O. and Tonning, F. M. (1986). Unilateral sensorineural hearing loss in children less than 15 years of age. *Scandinavian Audiology*, **15**, 131–7.

Hartvig Jensen, J., Johansen, P. A. and Borre, S. (1989a). Unilateral sensorineural hearing loss in children and auditory performance with respect to right/left ear differences. *British Journal of Audiology*, **23**, 207–14.

Hartvig Jensen, J., Borre, S. and Johansen, P. A. (1989b). Unilateral sensorineural hearing loss in children: cognitive abilities with respect to right/left ear differences. *British Journal of Audiology*, **23**, 215–20.

Moore, B. C. J. (1989). *An Introduction to the Psychology of Hearing*, 3rd edn London: Academic Press.

Newton, V. E. (1983). Sound localisation in children with severe unilateral hearing loss. *Audiology*, **22**, 189–98.

Tarkkanen, J. and Aho, J. (1966). Unilateral deafness in children. *Acta Otolaryngologica*, **61**, 270–81.

9

Management of sensorineural hearing loss

JACKIE MOON

Introduction

With the exception of cochlear implantation, sensorineural hearing loss cannot be corrected by surgical or medical treatment. Early and appropriate selection and use of amplification is important, therefore, for the hearing-impaired child. Hearing aids bring sound more effectively to the ear, they do not restore hearing to normal.

It is necessary to select a hearing aid that will provide maximum benefit for the individual on a consistent basis to help promote the development of language and communication skills. For congenitally deaf children better speech intelligibility is achieved if amplification is available within the first 6 months of life (Markides, 1986). Appropriate amplification makes an important contribution to the linguistic, social, intellectual and emotional development of a hearing-impaired child.

As a general guideline, amplification is required for hearing losses greater than 30 dB averaged across the speech frequency range 500–4000 Hz in the better ear. When amplification is indicated in very young hearing-impaired children, only limited information about a child's hearing sensitivity in this range is available, either from behavioural responses, using distraction testing or visual reinforcement audiometry, or from evoked response audiometry. The limitations of auditory brainstem response testing has already been described in Chapter 5.

It is essential that any child fitted with hearing aids is closely monitored and many clinic visits are required, particularly in the first year following hearing aid provision. In addition to audiological assessments in the clinic, hearing-impaired infants receive home visits from a specialist teacher of the deaf who provides guidance and support to the child's family. Observations from both parents and teachers are noted, and audiological assessment of the child is undertaken with and without hearing aids. The management of the child may be modified, with changes to the hearing aid prescription, as a more complete picture of their hearing sensitivity is obtained.

Components of a hearing aid

A hearing aid consists of a number of basic components: a microphone, amplifier, receiver and battery. These are shown in Figure 9.1. Incoming sound is converted to an electrical signal, which is amplified, converted to an acoustic signal, and delivered to the ear via the earmould. The life of a hearing aid battery depends upon several factors including the type of hearing aid, type of battery, hours of use and the required setting.

A volume or gain control, usually a numbered dial, adjusts the amount of amplification. Louder is not necessarily clearer, as sound is distorted when it is too loud. Parents are usually advised on the appropriate setting for their child. Another three position switch is normally available: O, off; M, microphone (on); and T, the telecoil position. The T position is used in conjunction with a loop installation, which enables the signal to be received directly without any background noise. A combined MT position is also found in some hearing aids, which includes both an environmental microphone and telecoil option to be used simultaneously.

A tone control may change the frequency response characteristic of the aid. Often it can reduce the low or high frequencies and is preset by the clinician. Methods of output limiting include peak clipping and

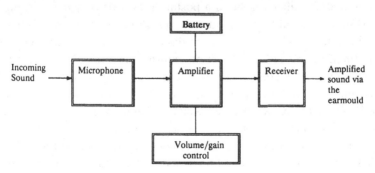

Figure 9.1. Block diagram of a basic hearing aid.

automatic gain control. These control the maximum output, the highest sound level that the aid can produce. It can 'compress' a range of sounds to fit within the user's reduced dynamic range of hearing. The dynamic range is the range between the threshold of hearing and the level at which the sound becomes uncomfortable, the loudness discomfort level.

Hearing aid systems have been discussed in detail by Pollack (1988) and Evans (1993).

Types of hearing aid systems
Conventional hearing aids

A number of types of hearing aid are available and these include postaural or behind-the-ear, intra-aural or in-the-ear, body-worn and bone-conduction aids.

Postaural aids are the most commonly fitted type and are worn behind the ear, coupled to the child's individual earmould as shown in Figures 9.2 and 9.3. Intra-aural aids fit into the canal and/or concha of the external ear, the components being mounted in the earmould.

Body-worn aids are usually worn in a harness on the child's chest. The receiver is clipped into the earmould and is connected to the aid by a lead. This is shown in Figure 9.4. Most hearing aids deliver the amplified acoustic signal to the external auditory meatus and then this amplified signal is transmitted through the middle ear to the cochlea. These systems work on an air-conduction principle.

In bone-conduction aids a vibratory signal is delivered to the cochlea from a head-worn receiver (the vibrator), which is placed on the mastoid bone. The signal is conveyed by bone/tissue vibration. The microphone and amplifier can be in a postaural or a body worn unit. Figure 9.5 shows a typical bone-conduction aid. Bone-conduction aids are fitted in cases of chronic infection, discharging ears or congenital ear abnormalities, including a narrow external meatus, atresia or absent pinna. Implanted bone-conduction aids now offer an alternative for children with bilateral atresia. Hakansson *et al.* (1985) have described the bone-anchored hearing aid, which is fitted by means of a titanium screw in the mastoid bone. The acoustic signal generated by a transducer is led to the skull by means of the percutaneous coupling.

Variations on postaural and bone-conduction aids include the spectacle aid in which the aid is incorporated into the frame. The signal can be

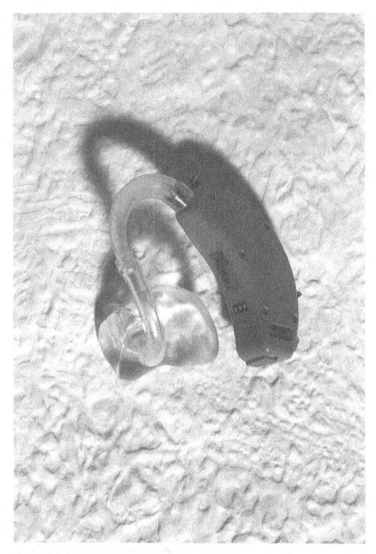

Figure 9.2. A mini postaural hearing aid and earmould.

delivered by a vibrator placed on the mastoid or by an earmould attached via an acoustic tube to a postaural aid. This is not commonly used in children, as it is not always a practical option.

A CROS aid (contralateral routing of signals) consists of a microphone and amplifier located at one ear and a receiver in the other. The two are usually linked by a flexible lead. This type of aid has been described in more detail by Evans (1993). It can be worn in cases of

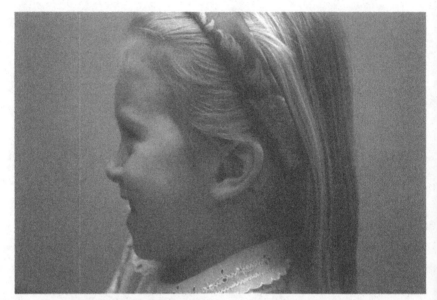

Figure 9.3. A mini postaural hearing aid and earmould in position.

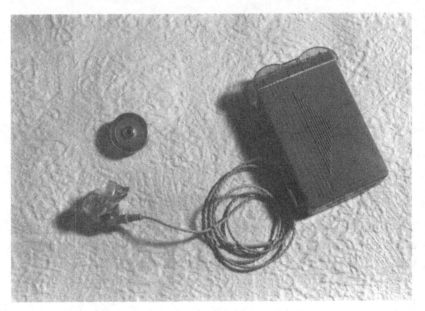

Figure 9.4. A body-worn aid with a separate receiver connected to the earmould.

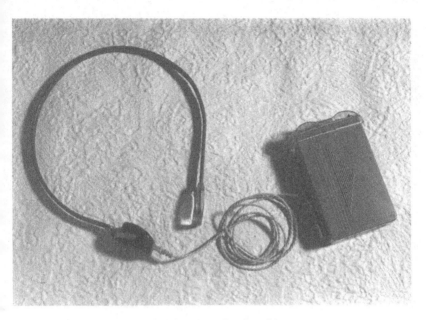

Figure 9.5. A typical bone-conduction aid.

unilateral loss or if there is an asymmetrical loss. A child with a severe unilateral hearing loss may, however, manage better without an aid. This is discussed in Chapter 8.

Alternative forms of personal aids

An alternative to conventional hearing aids for those who receive little benefit from amplification is a vibrotactile aid. These may be of some, although limited, benefit to profoundly deaf children. Acoustic information is presented to the wearer through vibrotactile stimulation (Figure 9.6). Tactile aids have been discussed in detail by Summers (1992).

Cochlear implants are another alternative for those who receive little benefit from conventional hearing aids. These are discussed further in Chapter 10.

Hearing aid selection

In selecting a hearing aid, consideration should be given to the gain of the aid and this should be chosen to suit the degree of hearing loss. The gain is the amount of amplification required. It is the difference

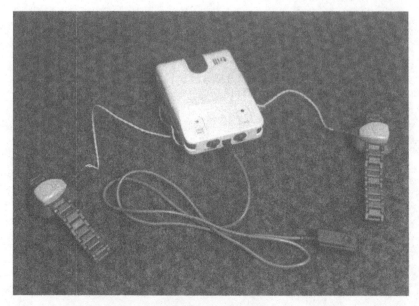

Figure 9.6. A vibrotactile aid in the form of a wrist-worn device that presents acoustic information to the wearer.

between the output and input sound levels, i.e. an input of 60 dBSPL giving an output of 110 dBSPL has 50 dB gain. The gain changes with frequency, resulting in a frequency response of the hearing aid as shown in Figure 9.7. The frequency response should be appropriate for the configuration of the hearing loss, e.g. if the child has a high frequency loss an aid with a high frequency emphasis is required.

A number of hearing aid selection procedures are available based on a prescription approach, e.g. Seewald *et al.* (1985) and Byrne and Dillon (1986). The limitation of these procedures is that hearing aids cannot be matched exactly to the prescription requirements. However, ergonomic factors, such as size, must be considered along with electroacoustic factors. The hearing aid fitting should always be evaluated. However, it takes a while for a child to make use of the improved sound signal received. Evaluation will give a measure of the amount of speech frequency information available to the child. It is important to ensure that adequate amplification is being used, while also avoiding high levels of amplification, which may be uncomfortable to the child and may result in rejection of the hearing aid.

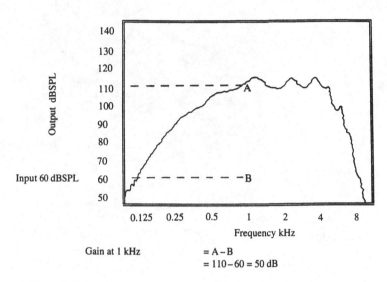

Figure 9.7. Basic frequency response of a hearing aid.

Earmoulds

The earmould directs amplified sound to the ear canal from the receiver. It is an integral part of the total electroacoustic system and it influences the amplified signal delivered to the individual. It is important that the earmould provides a good acoustic seal and is comfortable to wear. An impression is taken using a silicone material by a standard technique (BSA, 1987). This is shown in Figure 9.8. An appropriate soft material should be chosen, e.g. soft acrylic or molloplast, not only for the safety aspect, but also to enable high levels of gain and output to be delivered to severely and profoundly hearing-impaired children. Well fitting earmoulds are needed to prevent acoustic feedback – a high pitched whistle – which occurs when sound escapes and is re-amplified by the microphone. This feedback often prevents the use of optimum amplification.

Earmoulds need to be renewed on a regular basis in rapidly growing children, who require high amounts of gain. Feedback is a problem when the growth of the external meatus is rapid. Parents should not simply reduce the gain to reduce feedback, but should obtain new earmoulds to ensure that the aids are used to maximum effect.

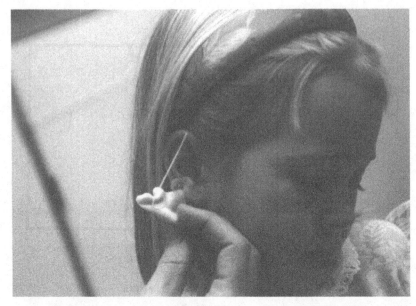

Figure 9.8. A silicone impression.

Advantages and limitations of hearing aid systems

The majority of children are fitted with postaural hearing aids and the general consensus is that a hearing aid should be fitted to each ear (a binaural fitting) unless there are any contraindications to this. Advantages of binaural fitting include an improvement in signal localisation and a summation effect, which results in higher signal levels. There is an improvement in hearing in background noise, i.e. improved signal detection in noise.

Conventional aids are not however able to pick up speech without also amplifying background noise. Remote microphone systems are available to optimise the signal in the presence of background noise and they help to overcome the signal-to-noise ratio problem. The advantages and limitations of these systems are discussed later in this chapter.

Postaural aids

Postaural hearing aids are now available with high gain and maximum output. They have the advantage of a more natural microphone position providing good localisation and good amplification close to the sound source. Small discreet and lightweight models are commercially available, although a mini low power postaural aid suitable for children is now included in the NHS range of hearing aids. The majority of NHS models are too big for tiny children. Figure 9.9 compares the size of mini and larger postaural hearing aids. Problems are experienced with the fitting of large hearing aids and sticky discs or plastic retainers may be required for secure placement. The drawback of mini aids is that the controls are less accessible and can be more difficult to manipulate.

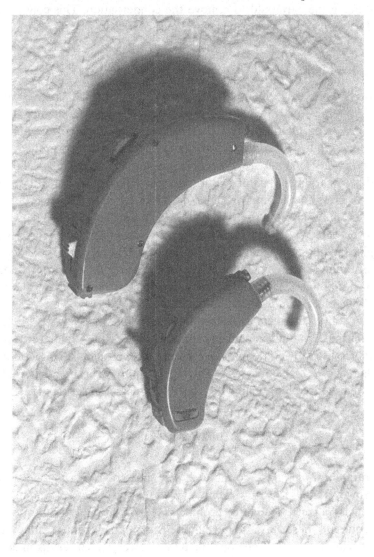

Figure 9.9. A mini and larger postaural hearing aid.

The majority of postaural aids do not have a battery indicator to warn of the voltage drop so it is necessary to change batteries regularly and check daily that the child's aid is functioning. A regular check must also be made for any blockage of the tubing. Condensation collects in the tubing as a result of the high humidity in the external auditory meatus. This can be removed by detaching the earmould from the aid and blowing air through the tubing using miniature bellows or simply by shaking the earmould to remove the condensation. This condensation, if excessive, can affect the performance of the aid.

Body-worn aids

Body-worn aids are usually securely positioned in a harness on the child's chest and the controls are larger and easier to manipulate than those on postaural instruments. These units are high powered and have a low frequency emphasis. This is of benefit to those severely deaf children who have only low frequency residual hearing. The availability of this low frequency information was the main advantage of body-worn aids prior to the improvement of postaural aids. The microphone is often fitted into the top of the aid, which enables the child's own voice to be detected. There are, however, disadvantages of this microphone placement on the child's chest, as the microphone can be shielded from incoming sounds by clothing. The response of the aid can be modified by both the body and the clothing, resulting in 'body-baffle'. The microphone placement is also vulnerable to spilt food.

Another disadvantage is the large and heavy receiver, which can prevent the earmould from fitting correctly in the ear. A miniature receiver can be used in an attempt to overcome this problem. A common fault is damage to the flexible lead. The lead can, however, be easily replaced. Children are able to alter the controls, unless a plastic cover is used to protect both the controls and the microphone.

Intra-aural aids

Intra-aural aids have cosmetic appeal and good microphone position. However, there are problems in that they are custom manufactured, which in turn leads to problems if post-fitting modifications are required. These aids also have limited gain and maximum output due to the closeness of the microphone and receiver, which results in acoustic feedback. They are usually suitable for mild–moderate hearing losses.

The controls are often inaccessible to parents and teachers. Intra-aural aids are generally not suitable for rapidly growing children, but may be appropriate for children with special requirements, such as those with a deformed pinna.

Bone-conduction aids

The signal is often distorted in bone-conduction aids due to the large mass of the transducer and the large amount of energy required to drive the bone vibrator. This results in a limited output of the system. There are also problems with comfort, positioning and lack of aesthetic appeal. Bone-conduction aids are usually fitted where only minimal gain is required and there is normal cochlear function, i.e. in cases of congenital conductive hearing loss. However, air-conduction fittings are usually preferred if clinically viable.

Remote microphone systems

There are several remote microphone systems including electromagnetic induction and radio aid systems. These two types are discussed briefly.

Electromagnetic induction – the loop system

In this system the input from the remote microphone is amplified and transmitted around an electromagnetic loop installed around a room, or around the child's neck. This system works in conjunction with the T position of the child's hearing aid. The use of this switch on the user control of a hearing aid has been discussed earlier in this chapter. The loop system is inexpensive and can overcome background noise, but is not usually the chosen system to be used in a classroom as it has many disadvantages. In the classroom a good teacher-to-child link is achieved, but there is not a child-to-child link unless there is a combined MT switch enabling an environmental microphone to be used. The system is prone to weak or dead spots with the strength of the signal varying with head position and orientation. There may be a spillover effect if two adjacent rooms are using the loop. Noise can also be picked up from other sources of electromagnetic radiation, e.g. fluorescent lighting. The gain of the hearing aid can also be reduced when set to receive the inductive signal. Loop systems are used mainly as assistive devices for television, telephone and in large public buildings including concert halls and churches.

Radio aid systems

Radio aids are the most popular type of remote microphone systems and are usually supplied by the local education service, although they are available on prescription from the hearing aid budget. They consist of a transmitter worn by the parent or teacher and a receiver worn by the child. The signal is delivered by frequency modulated (FM) radio transmission to the child's personal hearing aid. It has the advantage of overcoming the problem of background noise, improving the signal-to-noise ratio with the microphone positioned near to the preferred speaker. Radio aids usually have both an environmental microphone and an input from the FM receiver, which can be operated independently or in combination.

There are two types of radio aid. Type I is a body-worn aid worn as an FM system. In Type II radio aids the system is specifically set up to match each child's personal hearing aid and the signal is passed to the child's hearing aid via a lead using direct input or a neck loop. Direct input is a direct electrical connection between the radio receiver and hearing aid. This is shown in Figure 9.10. The majority of aids with a direct input facility are commercially available. However, the NHS has recently introduced a medium power aid with this facility (the BE36). These aids overcome the problem of background noise by transmitting the signal directly to the child's receiver. Type I has the advantage of there being less chance of feedback at high power. Type II enables the child to wear a personal aid, but eliminates the background noise. These systems work over a considerable distance and provide good amplification. Interference is not usually a problem and different transmission frequencies can be used, depending upon the activity of the child. One channel can be common to a group of children, while a child can have his or her own channel for one-to-one communication with the teacher. Different frequencies can be selected by changing the oscillator module. Five frequencies are currently designated for the use of radio hearing aid systems.

Rechargeable batteries are used and there is a visual indicator to warn that the battery needs replacement. These systems have the disadvantage of being expensive and being larger and more obvious than a conventional type of aid. If Type I aids are worn in school it is often necessary for the child to change to postaurals for use at home, resulting in a different quality of sound. The speaker must always remember to switch off the transmitter if talking to another child and the child-to-

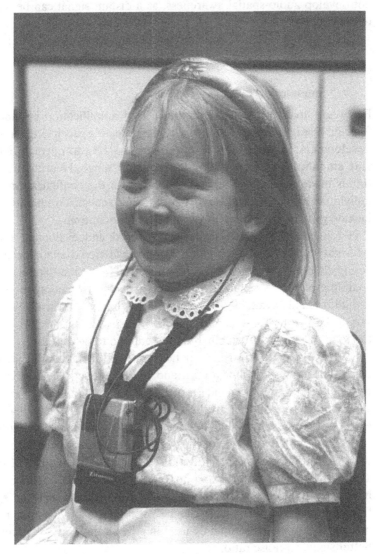

Figure 9.10. A Type II radio aid system in which the signal is passed from the body-worn radio receiver to the child's hearing aid via a lead.

child link in a classroom situation is poor, unless the combined environmental microphone is used. Radio aids have limited use at home as generally there are fewer competing speakers. There is a temptation to use the aid to communicate over a long distance, which would not be possible if a radio aid system was not available to the child. The wearer may not develop audio-spatial awareness, as a distant signal can be audible to the child.

Radio aid systems have been discussed in detail by Ross (1992).

Summary

Early and appropriate selection and use of amplification is important for the hearing-impaired child with regards to speech and language development. Hearing aids do not restore hearing to normal, but provide amplification across a limited frequency range. Hearing aid selection is made on a prescriptive basis, based on the configuration of the individual child's hearing loss. Chosen electroacoustic characteristics include gain, frequency response and maximum output.

Hearing aid fittings are closely monitored and evaluated. Limited information regarding a child's hearing sensitivity is available in very young children, which results in amplification being modified as a more complete picture is obtained. As much speech information as possible should be made available to the child using binaural hearing aids. This should be within the dynamic range of hearing, ensuring that it is not too loud to be uncomfortable, but loud enough to be useful.

Several types of conventional hearing aids are available including postaural, intra-aural, body-worn and bone-conduction. Basic components of a hearing aid include a microphone, amplifier and a receiver. The majority of children are fitted with postaural aids, and high powered ones are now available. Feedback is a common problem with high output aids, and it occurs when amplified sound escapes and is re-amplified. Well fitting earmoulds are required to avoid this leakage of sound. There are both advantages and limitations of all types of conventional hearing aids. The main limitation is that they cannot separate speech from background noise. This can be overcome by the use of remote microphone systems, commonly used in educational settings, enabling a better signal-to-noise ratio.

References

British Society of Audiology (1987). Recommended procedures for taking an aural impression. *British Journal of Audiology*, **20**, 315–17.

Byrne, D. and Dillon, H. (1986). The National Acoustic Laboratories (NAL) new procedures for selecting the gain and frequency response of a hearing aid. *Ear and Hearing*, **7**, 257–65.

Evans, P. I. P. (1993). Hearing aid systems. In *Paediatric Audiology 0–5 years*, 2nd edn (ed. B. McCormick), pp. 312–54. London: Whurr Publisher Limited.

Hakansson, B., Tjellstram, A., Rossenhall, V. and Carlsson, P. (1985). The bone anchored hearing aid. *Acta Otolaryngologica (Stockh.)*, **100**, 229–39.

Markides, A. (1986). Age at fitting of hearing aids and speech intelligibility. *British Journal of Audiology*, **20**, 165–8.

Pollack, M. C. (1988). Electroacoustic characteristics. In *Amplification for the Hearing Impaired*, 3rd edn (ed. M. C. Pollack), pp. 21–103. New York: Grune and Stratton.

Ross, M. (ed.) (1992). *F.M. Auditory Training Systems. Characteristics, Selection and Use*. Timonium, Maryland: York Press.

Seewald, R. C., Ross, M. and Spiro, M. K. (1985). Selecting amplification characteristics for young hearing impaired children. *Ear and Hearing*, **6**, 48–53.

Seewald, R. C. and Ross, M. (1988). Amplification for young hearing impaired children. In *Amplification for the Hearing Impaired*, 3rd edn (ed. M. C. Pollack), pp. 213–71. New York: Grune and Stratton.

Summers, I. R. (ed.) (1992). *Tactile Aids for the Hearing Impaired*. London: Whurr Publishers Limited.

10
Cochlear implants

SARAH SHEPPARD

Introduction

Cochlear implants are a relatively new form of assistive device for the profoundly deaf who receive little, if any, benefit from the conventional acoustic hearing aids described in Chapter 9. Of the one per thousand children who have profound hearing loss only a very small proportion will be sufficiently deaf to require a cochlear implant. For this small group cochlear implants can provide access to auditory forms of communication and thus help to promote the child's social, emotional and educational development. The function of cochlear implants is to bypass non-functional or absent structures in the cochlea and stimulate the remaining auditory nerve fibres by direct electrical stimulation. The electrically induced nerve impulses are transmitted to the auditory centres of the brain to produce a sensation of hearing (Figure 10.1).

Initially only adults with acquired hearing losses were selected for implantation but since significant benefit from implantation in adults has been demonstrated, considerable numbers of children have been implanted, including young congenitally deaf children. There has been resistance to implantation worldwide, partly because of fears of long term adverse effects of implantation, which have so far not materialised, and also because implantation has been wrongly perceived as a cure for profound deafness rather than as another assistive device.

Cochlear implant design

Hardware

Cochlear implant systems vary in their design but have several common components. Externally there is a microphone, which picks up sound and converts it into an electrical signal, which is then modified by a

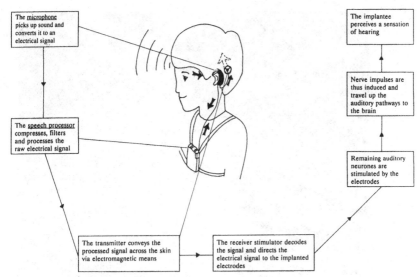

Figure 10.1. Flow diagrams of how the different components of a cochlear implant system function to induce a sensation of hearing.

speech processor into a form suitable to be delivered to the internal implanted receiver/stimulator and electrode array (Figure 10.2). The processed signal may be transmitted from the external components of the system to the implanted electrodes either transcutaneously, that is across the skin by electromagnetic means, or percutaneously via a plug through the skin. Transcutaneous systems have the disadvantage that new developments in implant design may be more difficult to implement but most paediatric programmes prefer transcutaneous links because of the increased risk of damage and infection around the plug of percutaneous systems. Usually the microphone, speech processor and transmitter coil are separate units connected by cables but there is now one system in which the microphone and speech processor are housed in the same case worn behind the ear.

Electrode number and position

To create an electric field to stimulate neural tissue, electric current must flow between an active and a reference or ground electrode. Cochlear implants therefore require at least one active and one reference electrode and may be described as extracochlear or intracochlear depending on the site of the active electrodes. Extracochlear electrodes are placed on the promontory or round window, thus causing no

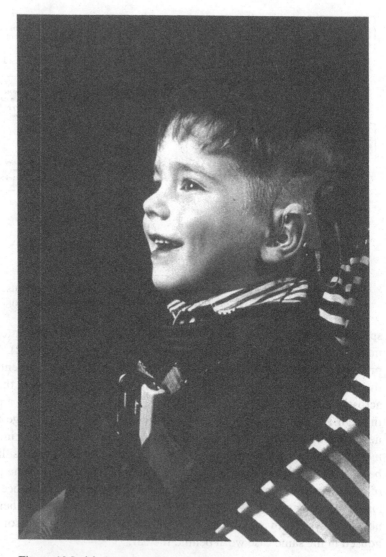

Figure 10.2. (a) A young child wearing the external components of a cochlear implant system.

damage to the cochlea but resulting in the signal being delivered further away from the auditory nerve endings. Intracochlear placement of electrodes necessitates the surgeon drilling into the cochlea to insert the electrode array, thus causing some disruption to the remaining structures but allowing stimulation closer to the auditory nerve tissue. Some

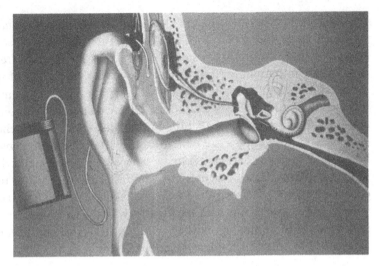

Figure 10.2. (b) The external and internal parts of the cochlear implant system.

implant systems are single-channel, using only one active electrode, whereas multi-channel systems have several active electrodes through which different information is conveyed. It is generally accepted that intracochlear multi-channel systems produce the best results although very good results have been occasionally obtained with some single-channel implantees.

Speech processing

Some form of signal or speech processing is carried out by the speech processor of all implant systems so that as much of the auditory stimulus as possible is represented to the implantee. For a normally hearing ear there is a very broad range between sounds that are just audible and sound levels that are so loud as to be uncomfortable. This range is referred to as the acoustic dynamic range. The dynamic range for electrical stimulation used to evoke a sensation of hearing is very small and the normal range must be 'squashed' into the reduced electrical dynamic range. If the electrical stimulus is too low no sound will be perceived but if electrical stimulation is too high the implantee will experience pain. Different cochlear implant systems employ different methods of speech processing, which is roughly comparable to different software being used to operate different types of computer. The electric current may be presented to the electrodes as a continuous analogue waveform or as a series of short, fast pulses. The speech processor may also emphasise certain features of speech such as the formant frequencies that are important for discriminating speech. Other types of speech processor select different frequency bands of the auditory signal and transmit them to different electrodes. Single-channel devices compress and filter the signal but send all the information via the same channel. New and more complex speech processing strategies are constantly being developed for existing and new devices. Continuous interleaved sampling utilises pulsatile signals at a very fast sampling rate, to try and conserve timing features of speech and avoid channel interactions, which can be a problem with analogue devices. Other new strategies look at ways of improving existing pulsatile strategies and developing combined pulsatile and continuous analogue strategies.

Implant systems used with children

There are now several different types of implant systems available either clinically or still at the research and development stage. A significant number of children in the USA were implanted with House's first clinical device, which was a single-channel device. At the present time however most implanted children have Nucleus 22 Multi-channel cochlear implants. The Nucleus device has been used extensively with adults and is currently the only implant system that has full approval of the USA Food and Drug Administration (FDA) for use with children. Children's demands of an implant system, in terms of safety and durability as well as the quality of the sound sensation induced, can be considered to be greater than adults because they are likely to use the device for a longer period of time and will be developing speech and language rather than reawakening spoken language learnt previously.

The cochlear implant team

Worldwide team approaches to implantation have produced the best results for patients. A team for children should involve a core of medical, audiological and rehabilitation personnel, usually otologists, audiological scientists, teachers of the deaf and speech and language therapists who are experienced in working with the paediatric population. All team members need to function interactively, and have their own input into the management of patients throughout the assessment,

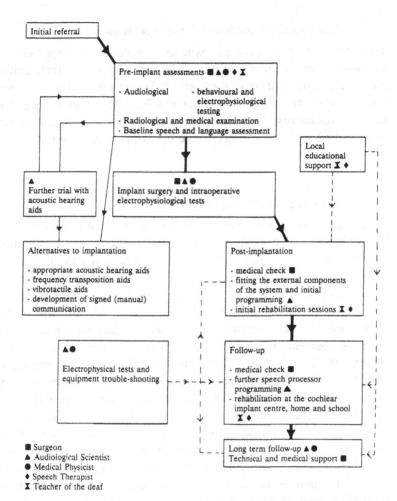

Figure 10.3. A schedule for assessment, implantation and rehabilitation showing the involvement of different cochlear implant team members.

implantation and rehabilitation phases (Figure 10.3). The team should provide a cohesive service with appropriate facilities and techniques for children. A solid foundation of knowledge about general paediatric audiology is very beneficial at all stages of the implantation process but also in being able to discuss and arrange alternative help and support for children who for some reason do not go ahead with implantation.

Assessment of candidates for implantation

Implantation is an invasive and expensive procedure that requires considerable commitment on the part of implanted children, their families and teachers, in addition to the team at the implant centre. It is therefore necessary to ensure that other less invasive forms of help have been exhausted first. The child must be assessed audiologically, medically and educationally to determine his or her suitability for cochlear implantation.

Audiological assessment

Audiological assessment involves evaluating the child's response to frequency-specific auditory stimuli with and without hearing aids to determine the degree of benefit afforded by the aids using the behavioural techniques discussed in Chapter 3. Ideally the child should be mature enough to carry out the performance type of test technique, which is also used for programming the speech processor after implantation. Distraction testing and visual reinforcement audiometry may be used during assessment but cannot sustain the child's interest long enough to produce the large number of responses required for programming the speech processor of multichannel devices. In practice, implantation is not generally recommended under the age of 2 years because of the difficulty in obtaining enough accurate audiological information and also because of possible surgical complications that may arise owing to rapid skull growth below the age of 2 years. Prior to carrying out this assessment it is important to exclude any treatable component to the hearing loss, such as middle-ear fluid, by otological examination and middle-ear impedance measurements. The child's hearing aids should be checked to ensure that they are functioning correctly and should be the most appropriate for the child's hearing loss. Electrophysiological tests, usually auditory brainstem electric response testing (Chapter 5), are carried out to confirm the degree of hearing loss objectively. If there is any residual response present it may be possible to obtain some information about whether the hearing loss originates in the cochlea or higher up the auditory pathway. The absence of evoked otoacoustic emissions (Chapter 5) is indicative of cochlear dysfunction but does not exclude some neural component to the hearing loss. The presence of otoacoustic emissions indicates that the cochlea is functioning and that any hearing loss may be neural in origin and possibly not amenable to implantation. It is not, however, clear how much surviving auditory neural tissue is necessary for a cochlear implant to provide benefit, although individuals later found to have degeneration of auditory nerve endings have performed well with implants. There is no test available that will give conclusive information about the condition of auditory nerve endings in a hearing-impaired person. Preimplant stimulation of the promontory or round window has been used with adults and gives some information but a negative result is not necessarily a contraindication for implantation. This sort of test is invasive and unsuitable for children. In the future it may be possible to further refine electrophysiological tests for this purpose. If a child receives no significant benefit from suitable conventional aids after an extended trial period of several months use, and this is confirmed by audiological assessment, other investigations of suitability for implantation may proceed. It is often necessary for young children to be seen at the cochlear implant centre several times to complete audiological and electrophysiological measurements.

Medical and radiological investigations

Medical and radiological assessments are needed firstly to ensure that the child is fit enough to undergo surgery and secondly to check that the cochlea is patent, and to look for any deformity in the cochlea. Usually computerised tomography (CT) scanning is used but as magnetic resonance imaging (MRI) becomes more refined this may become the preferred imaging technique. It is important to note that cochlear implants, when fitted, often prevent the use of MRI because of the implanted magnet and metallic components. If the cochlea is found to be ossified, as is frequently the case after meningitis, or if there is a deformity of the cochlea, the surgeon needs to assess whether implantation within the cochlea is possible at all or whether a single-channel extracochlear device is preferable. Time should be allocated for discussion of any risk of implantation since many parents are anxious about the surgery. Ethical issues surrounding the decision to go ahead with implantation should also be considered. With young children parents often have to make medical decisions on behalf of their children. For children deafened when they are young, early implantation produces optimum results; if implantation is delayed until the child is older it is possible that good results will no longer be achievable. Parents therefore need clear and comprehensive information to make the decision to implant on behalf of their children.

Educational assessment

Baseline information about the child's speech and language status before implantation is important in planning effective rehabilitation and in assessing progress in speech and language development after implantation. Useful information about the child's use of hearing aids can support audiological assessment at this stage.

Throughout the assessment process it is important that parents and children are given ample time to discuss all aspects of implantation with whichever member of the implant team they wish to, so that they can make an informed decision on whether to go ahead with implantation. The team can be there to provide information and support but the child's family must make the decision as to whether their child is implanted, if all of the assessments are satisfactory.

Surgery

The surgery required to insert the electrode array and the receiver/stimulator varies according to which device is used. Children are usually admitted to hospital for 4 to 5 days. After administration of a general anaesthetic the hair is shaved above and behind the ear to be implanted. An incision in the shape of a C or U is made behind the ear, creating a fairly large skin flap so that sutures are remote from the receiver/stimulator package, thus minimising the risk of skin flap infections. The mastoid bone is drilled to form a cavity to gain access to the cochlea and a bed is created in the skull in which to seat the receiver/stimulator. Intracochlear devices are inserted gently into the scala tympani via the round window niche, which may have been enlarged slightly by drilling, or via a hole drilled in the bone directly over the scala tympani. Ideally the whole electrode array is inserted but sometimes there is some ossification of soft tissue, which may impede complete insertion. It is still possible to gain significant benefit from partial insertion although if only very few electrodes can be inserted into the cochlea some surgeons prefer to use a single-channel device extracochlearly in the round window niche or on the surface of the promontory. The receiver/stimulator is secured in position with Dacron ties and a bulky pressure dressing is applied to the wound after suturing. Towards the end of the implant operation it is possible to carry out intraoperative tests of implant function. The results of these tests are very useful in the subsequent fitting and tuning or programming of the external parts of the implant system for children. Two techniques can be used to elicit an auditory response by stimulating the implant. The stapedial reflex (Chapter 6) and the auditory brainstem response (Chapter 5) can be elicited with electrical stimulation via the implant and are known as the ESRT (electrical stapedial reflex threshold) and the EABR (electrical auditory brainstem response).

As with any surgical procedure, there are occasional complications. These may include facial nerve stimulation, which may resolve spontaneously or by changing the programming of the electrodes involved, skin flap infections, balance or taste disturbances. A case of meningitis following implant surgery has been reported. Occasionally the internal device itself may fail or be rejected but successful reimplantations of similar and in some cases different implants have been achieved.

Fitting and programming the speech processor

The external components of the implant system: the speech processor, microphone and transmitter coil, are usually fitted 3 to 4 weeks after implantation when the child has fully recovered from surgery. It is often helpful for the child to have the opportunity to see and handle the external equipment prior to the first programming session so that he or she becomes familiar with the equipment. The programming or tuning of the speech processor involves carrying out measurements that enable the clinician to adjust processor settings to match each individual's dynamic range for electrical stimulation. Threshold measurements, that is the level at which stimulation through the implant is just audible, and maximum comfortable loudness levels are measured for each electrode channel for multichannel devices and at different frequencies for single-channel broad band devices.

Threshold measurements are usually carried out using conditioned responses to sound stimulation as described for the performance test in Chapter 3. Most implanted children will have had little if any prior experience of sound and therefore conditioning may have to be re-established using vibrotactile or visual stimulation first. The results of EABR measurements carried out intraoperatively can be invaluable during the early stages of threshold measurements.

Children need to be seen frequently after initial stimulation to check previous measurements and to proceed further with introducing new electrodes and increasing the dynamic range gradually. The functioning and condition of the external equipment of the implant system will need

122   *S. Sheppard*

to be checked at follow-up sessions because children are not necessarily able to indicate if there is a problem with their implant system. Teachers and parents need to be vigilant to any changes in the child's responsiveness or behaviour, which may indicate that the child is receiving a poor signal or none at all through the implant.

The child's progress with the implant can be assessed in the clinic using standard techniques for paediatric audiology as described in Chapters 3 and 9. Sound field warble tone measurements using the performance technique with the child using his or her implant system can give an indication of the level at which different frequencies of sound are heard, although results are influenced by the internal and user settings of the speech processor and should be interpreted with caution. With substantial experience using their implant systems, children may be able to carry out simple speech discrimination tests with, and later without, lipreading such as the McCormick Toy Discrimination Test and the automated version of this test described in Chapter 3 (Figure 10.4). Measurements carried out in the clinic can be supplemented by feedback from rehabilitation activities carried out at the implant centre and in the child's own school and home settings.

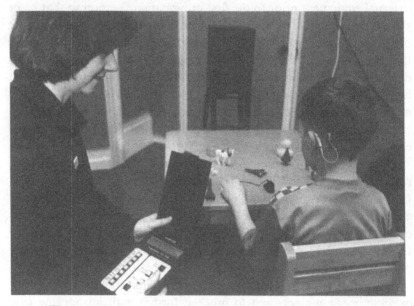

Figure 10.4. A young child using his cochlear implant to carry out speech discrimination testing with the automated McCormick Toy Discrimination Test.

Rehabilitation

This is the process of helping the child to use the auditory signals received through the implant to the maximum potential. The rehabilitation techniques need to be adapted to suit individual children. Progress may appear slow to parents, especially during the first 6 months after implantation, but discussion with teachers of the deaf and speech and language therapists about changes in their child's functioning with the implant can provide considerable encouragement to parents and the application of appropriate rehabilitation procedures is vital.

Results and benefits following implantation

Cochlear implants have now been used for significant periods of time by adults and children, with the result that most implantees' lives have changed considerably following implantation. Some multi-channel implant users are able to carry out limited conversations on the telephone. Children previously showing no awareness of sound have, following implantation, become aware of speech and environmental sounds and later been able to understand speech to a considerable degree without lipreading. Studies show that multi-channel implantees generally perform better at speech discrimination tasks than implantees who used the earlier single-channel implants. There is, however, a wide range in the individual performance of implantees, which is thought to be due to a variety of factors such as age, duration of deafness, type of implant, degree of neuronal survival and cooperation of the implantee and the family with device programming and rehabilitation. Probably the most important benefit of implantation is improved speech production and perception ability. Improvements in speech perception in implanted children is now well documented, with significant proportions of implanted children able to carry out speech discrimination tests without the aid of lipreading. Implanted children also show improvements in varying degrees in their ability to produce speech. Implantees' performance compares well with successful users of conventional hearing aids. Many adults have reached their maximum level of performance with their implants within 6 months to a year of implant use but children may still show improvements in their performance for several years after implantation, such that it is not yet possible to know the full benefits of implanting young deaf children. As better results from children become evident the criteria for implantation may be relaxed to include those children who receive some but marginal benefit from conventional aids as well as those who receive no benefit.

Summary

Cochlear implantation provides a relatively new form of help for profoundly hearing-impaired children who are not able to benefit from conventional acoustic hearing aids. Cochlear implants function by converting and processing an acoustic signal into an electrical signal that bypasses damaged or absent structures in the cochlea and stimulates remaining auditory neurones directly, thus giving a sensation of hearing. Detailed assessment of candidates' suitability for implantation is advisable, to ensure that other forms of help have been exhausted and to check that there are no contraindications to implantation. Cochlear implants comprise several components worn externally and an internal electrode array, which is surgically implanted. The implant does not restore normal hearing and implantees are still 'deaf' when external components of the system are not in use. In order to achieve the best signal the speech processor of the implant system has to be programmed to suit each individual implantee. For this signal to be interpreted optimally by the implantee extensive rehabilitation is required. Implanted children require specialised techniques and methods for device programming and rehabilitation, which are best carried out by professionals experienced at working with young deaf children. Paediatric implantation should therefore be regarded in terms of a programme of assessment, implantation, device programming and rehabilitation, which may extend over a period of years. The best results are obtained using a team of different professions working together to provide a cohesive, paediatrically oriented service. Cochlear implantation is an expensive and invasive procedure but when carried out in the context of an appropriately staffed paediatric programme can produce tremendous benefits for children who previously had no access to auditory stimulation or auditory means of communication.

Further reading

American Journal of Otology (1991). Supplement 12, Cochlear Implants in Children.

Clark, G. M., Tong, Y. C. and Patrick, J. F. (eds.) (1990). *Cochlear Prostheses*. London: Churchill Livingstone.

Cohen, N. L. and Hoffman, R. A. (1991). Complications of cochlear implant surgery in adults and children. *Annals of Otology, Rhinology, Laryngology*, **100**, 708–11.

Cooper, H. (ed.) (1991). *Cochlear Implants – a Practical Guide*. London: Whurr Publishers Limited.

Harnsberger, H. R., Dart, D. J., Parkin, J. L., Smoker, W. R. K. and Osborn, A. G. (1987). Cochlear implant candidates: assessments with CT and MR imaging, *Radiology*, **164**, 53–7.

McCormick, B. (1991). Paediatric cochlear implantation in the United Kingdom – a delayed journey on a well marked route. *British Journal of Audiology*, **25**, 145–9.

McCormick, B., Archbold, S. M. and Sheppard, S. (1994). *Cochlear Implants in Young Children*. London: Whurr Publishers Limited.

Parisier, S. C., Chute, P. M., Weiss, M. H., Hellman, S. A. and Wang, R. C. (1991). Results of cochlear implant reinsertions, *Laryngoscope*, **101**, 1013–15.

Sheppard, S. (1993). Cochlear implants. In *Paediatric Audiology, 0–5 years* (ed. B. McCormick), pp. 402–36. London: Whurr Publishers Limited.

Tucci, D. L., Lambert, P. R. and Ruth, R. A. (1990). Trends in rehabilitation after cochlear implantation. *Archives of Otolaryngology, Head and Neck Surgery*, **116**, 571–4.

Tyler, R. S. (ed.) (1993). *Cochlear implants, Audiological Foundations*. London: Whurr Publishers Limited.

Index

hearing loss
  causes, 8–15
    see also causes of deafness
  effect of grommets, 84
  and otitis media with effusion, 78
  history, 78–9
    see also otitis media with effusion
  unilateral, 87–95
    aetiology, 87
    assessment, 89
    effects, 88–9
    management, 89–94
      amplification, 93
      classroom seating, 90–2
      hearing conservation, 93–4
      hearing tactics, 90
      road safety, 93
    prevalence, 87
    psychoacoustic advantages of binaural
      hearing, 87–8
    psychoacoustic phenomena, 88
high tone sensorineural deafness,
    inconsistency of input, 4–5
high tone test stimulus, 5
House's first cochlear implant, 116
hysterical conversion deafness,
    investigating, 5

IHR/McCormick Automated Toy
    Discrimination Test, 28–9
immitance, definition, 67
immitance meters, 66
impedance
  definition, 67
  measurements, 17
impedance meters, 66
incubator noise, effect on neonatal
    cochlea, 11
infants hearing tests, 7
infection, and nasal obstruction, 82–3
inner ear, developmental abnormalities, 10
  causing deafness, 10
intensity of pure tone audiometry, 32
intra-aural aids, advantages and
    limitations, 106–7
intracranial haemorrhage, cause of
    deafness, 11

kernicterus as cause of deafness, 9
Klippel–Feil syndrome, deafness
    associated with, 10–11

language difficulties, delays or disorders,
    performance test, 24–5
loop system, 107
  advantages and disadvantages, 107
low birth weight preterm infants, deafness

  associated with, 11

magnetic resonance imaging
  before cochlear implantation, 119
  cochlear implants prevent use, 119
masking in pure tone audiometry, 39
  British Society of Audiology procedures,
    39
  cross–masking, 39
  examples, 39–47
  masked threshold measurement, 39
  use with children, 47–8
maternal infection during pregnancy as
    cause of deafness, 9
meningitis
  cause of acquired sensorineural
    deafness, 11–12
  as cause for hearing loss, 1
middle ear
  bleeding into, causing conductive
    deafness, 14
  see also otitis media: otitis media with
    effusion
middle-ear analysers, 66
middle-ear cleft, developmental
    abnormalities, 10
  causing deafness, 10
middle-ear effusion, 73
  see also otitis media: otitis media with
    effusion
middle-ear impedance, underlying
    principles, 65–6
middle-ear measurements, 65–74
  acoustic reflex decay, 72–3
  acoustic reflex threshold, 72
  middle-ear effusion, 73
  middle-ear stapedial reflex
    measurements, 72
  need, 65
  systems, 66–7
  terminology, 67
  tympanometry, 67–72
    see also tympanometry
middle ear in tympanometry
  compliance, 68, 70
  pressure, 68, 70
  volume, 68–9, 70
Mondini dysplasia of the cochlea causing
    deafness, 10
mucositis, middle ear, cause of conductive
    deafness, 12
myringotomy, 84

nasal obstruction and otitis media with
    effusion, 82–3
Neisseria meningitidis as cause of deafness,
    12

Printed in the United States
By Bookmasters